Epidemiology and Culture

This book shows how practitioners in the emerging field of "cultural epidemiology" describe human health, communicate with diverse audiences, and intervene to improve health and prevent disease. It uses textual and statistical portraits of disease to describe past and present collaborations between anthropology and epidemiology. Interpreting epidemiology as a cultural practice helps to reveal the ways in which measurement, causal thinking, and intervention design are all influenced by belief, habit, and theories of power. By "unpacking" many common disease risks and epidemiologic categories, this book reveals unexamined assumptions and shows how sociocultural context influences measurement of disease. Examples include studies of epilepsy, cholera, mortality on the *Titanic*, breastfeeding, and adolescent smoking. The book describes methods as varied as observing individuals, measuring social networks, and compiling data from death certificates. It argues that effective public health interventions must work more often and better at the level of entire communities.

JAMES A. TROSTLE is Associate Professor of Anthropology and Director of Urban Initiatives at Trinity College, Hartford. He has worked in more than 20 countries during his career in international health, and he has been invited to lecture in many others. He has co-authored, in Spanish, *De la Investigación en Salud a la Política: La Difícil Traducción (From Health Research to Policy: The Difficult Translation)*. He has published in *Health, Policy and Planning; Neurology; The Annual Review of Anthropology; Culture, Medicine and Psychiatry; Medical Anthropology Quarterly;* and, most frequently, in *Social Science and Medicine.* Professor Trostle has been a Temporary Advisor to the World Health Organization, and currently he sits on a WHO Task Force on Research to Policy as well as on the WHO Human Reproduction Programme Regional Advisory Panel for the Americas.

Cambridge Studies in Medical Anthropology

Editor

ALAN HARWOOD *University of Massachusetts, Boston*

Editorial Board

WILLIAM DRESSLER *University of Alabama*
RONALD FRANKENBERG *Brunel University, UK*
MARY JO GOOD *Harvard University*
SHARON KAUFMAN *University of California, San Francisco*
SHIRLEY LINDENBAUM *City University of New York*
MARGARET LOCK *McGill University*
CATHERINE PANTER-BRICK *University of Durham, UK*

Medical Anthropology is the fastest-growing specialist area within anthropology, both in North America and in Europe. Beginning as an applied field serving public health specialists, medical anthropology now provides a significant forum for many of the most urgent debates in anthropology and the humanities. It includes the study of medical institutions and health care in a variety of rich and poor societies, the investigation of the cultural construction of illness, and the analysis of ideas about the body, birth, maturity, ageing, and death.

This series includes theoretically innovative monographs, state-of-the-art collections of essays on current issues, and short books introducing main themes in the subdiscipline.

Epidemiology and Culture

James A. Trostle
Trinity College, Hartford

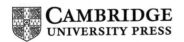

CAMBRIDGE
UNIVERSITY PRESS

CAMBRIDGE UNIVERSITY PRESS
Cambridge, New York, Melbourne, Madrid, Cape Town, Singapore, São Paulo

Cambridge University Press
40 West 20th Street, New York, NY 10011-4211, USA

www.cambridge.org
Information on this title: www.cambridge.org/9780521790505

First published 2005

Printed in the United States of America

A catalog record for this book is available from the British Library.

Library of Congress Cataloging in Publication data

Trostle, James A., 1954–
Epidemiology and culture / by James A. Trostle
    p. cm. – (Cambridge studies in medical anthropology ; 13)
Includes bibliographical references and index.
ISBN 0-521-79050-6 – ISBN 0-521-79389-0 (pbk.)
1. Epidemiology. 2. Medical anthropology. I. Title. II. Series.
RA652.T76   2004
614.4–dc22   2004051869

ISBN-13   978-0-521-79050-5 hardback
ISBN-10   0-521-79050-6 hardback

ISBN-13   978-0-521-79389-6 paperback
ISBN-10   0-521-79389-0 paperback

Contents

Figures and Tables

Figures

Tables

Foreword

I have been waiting to read this book for 20 years. In 1983, I had a student in one of my classes at Berkeley, a young man named Jim Trostle, who challenged almost everything I said. Trostle was at the time a doctoral student in the Medical Anthropology program at Berkeley (a joint program with the Medical School in San Francisco), and he had taken off a year to get a Masters of Public Health degree. I was a Professor of Social Epidemiology in the School of Public Health, and my research and teaching involved the study of psychosocial factors as they influenced the causation of disease. Trostle argued that I was not paying enough attention to the concept of culture and that my research would suffer as a result. He said that epidemiologists and anthropologists had to find a way to work together so that both could be more effective contributors to human welfare.

I thought he might be right, but it was too difficult an idea to take seriously. Epidemiologists use quantitative methods in studies of large populations, whereas anthropologists do qualitative, ethnographic studies in remote Pacific islands. We read different books, we use a different language, and we have very different intellectual histories and traditions. Nevertheless, here was Trostle in my class, learning the new language and trying to find a way to bridge the gap between us. I didn't know if he could accomplish this difficult feat, but I was betting against it.

Since that time, we epidemiologists have suffered a whole series of very embarrassing failures. We had been doing our research attempting to identify disease risk factors. That is what epidemiologists do. But the reason for this type of research is to help people lower their rate of disease. Our model is to identify the risk factors and share that information with a waiting public so that they will then rush home and, in the interests of good health, change their behaviors to lower their risk. It is a reasonable model, but it hasn't worked. In intervention study after intervention study, people have been informed about the things they need to do, and they have failed to follow our advice.

For example, in California, the State Health Department has for the last 15 years made it a major priority to inform people about the importance of eating five fruits and vegetables a day. Over the course of these 15 years, surveys of representative samples of the population have clearly shown that people understand the message. These same surveys, however, also show no change at all in eating behavior. There has been no increase in the frequency of fruits and vegetables in diets. The only thing that has increased during this time is obesity.

I myself have devoted enormous amounts of time and energy in the design and conduct of superb intervention studies. These studies were brilliant in conception, and they were implemented as well as any studies could be. All failed to produce their intended result. After many years of brooding, I have finally come to an opinion about one reason for this: We in public health have important messages to give to people, but people have lives to lead. There often is a major gap between these two priorities. This is an issue that anthropologists think about, and it would be good to incorporate that thinking into the design of better interventions.

I have come to another conclusion: I decided that Trostle had been right all along, and I hoped that one day he would write a book about the issue. This book comes none too soon. We all know that our medical care system is at a very strained point. The baby boomer population in the United States will enter the over-65-year-old group very soon (between 2020 and 2030), and when they do, the number of old people in the United States population will have doubled. If we think the medical care system is in difficulty now, we ain't seen nothin' yet. We must learn how to prevent disease in the first place and not simply wait until people are already sick. To develop effective interventions, epidemiology must learn how to understand the concept of culture, and epidemiologists must learn how to work with anthropologists as partners. And anthropologists must learn to work with epidemiologists as partners. This book goes a long way toward making this a realistic possibility.

In addition to the crucial issues discussed in this important book, attention must be given to the way in which both anthropologists and epidemiologists define such issues as health and illness and suffering. As long as the focus of our work is limited to specific diseases (asthma, coronary heart disease) and disease-specific risk factors (obesity, cholesterol), our research will always be removed from many of the things that people care about in their everyday lives, such as their jobs, children, debts, family, and happiness. It is important that both anthropologists and epidemiologists find ways to focus their research on these fundamental determinants of disease susceptibility.

For example, we are now doing an intervention among fifth graders living in a low-income community in California. The grant we received to do this work was intended to influence smoking and other drug use among these children as well as violence and school performance. But we are in fact intervening on the culture of hope. If these children believe they will be dead by the age of 20, it really does not matter much if they smoke or do badly in school. Hope, on the other hand, is something they care about, and if we are successful, the results might influence smoking, drugs, school behavior, and many other health-related issues. In another study, we are observing a large group of bus drivers who have high rates of hypertension, back trouble, gastrointestinal complaints, respiratory difficulties, and alcohol problems. We could (and should) deal with each problem, but we also must learn to focus on the fundamental and underlying determinant of all of these problems: the culture of the job itself. This is an issue that the drivers care about deeply.

The effort to identify fundamental problems that people care about and that also influence rates of health and illness is one that requires a partnership between anthropologists and epidemiologists. If these two groups could find a way to collaborate, we hopefully could design more effective and meaningful interventions.

This book lays out the principles necessary to help this process along. It is a courageous and visionary book. It has taken me many years to understand the wisdom of Jim Trostle's views, and I am pleased that now a whole group of new people all over the world will be exposed to them.

S. Leonard Syme, Professor Emeritus
University of California, Berkeley

Acknowledgments

In 1978 an anthropology professor at Columbia University, Ida Susser, told me that she was enrolled in a postdoctoral training program in "psychiatric epidemiology" at Columbia's medical school. As a naive undergraduate I thought it alarming – and wonderful – that one could study a field that contained so many syllables. My anthropological training at Columbia under Lambros Comitas, Alexander Alland, Charles Harrington, Marvin Harris, Leith Mullings, Joan Vincent, Ida Susser, and George Bond enabled me to build larger pictures out of the fine-grained details of individual observations and interviews. Anthropology provided ways to understand the variability, context, and rationales for health-related practices. I hoped epidemiology would give me theories and tools to understand the frequency and correlates of such practices. As I learned more, I found epidemiology to be a powerful strategy for describing health-related social problems at scale, summarizing multiple disease occurrences into patterns and flows, and looking for broad causes without descending into individual accounts.

I took up a series of paid internships, summer jobs, and, eventually, fulltime employment at the Sergievsky Center, an epidemiological research institute at Columbia's College of Physicians and Surgeons. Al Hauser and Mervyn Susser gave me good training and real responsibilities, and I will be forever grateful to both of them. At Sergievsky, Gerry Oppenheimer, Richard Neugebauer, and Ruth Ottman encouraged and answered my naive questions. Len Syme at University of California, Berkeley, and Fred Dunn at University of California, San Francisco, were my primary mentors during my doctoral training. I could not have done better than to find them both. And Al Hauser, Len Kurland, and Frank Sharbrough helped my doctoral research find its way through the Mayo Clinic bureaucracy, seven committees deep.

As I continued to mix anthropological and epidemiological methods I became passionate about finding others who had explored these disciplines before me. During library work and interviews in Los Angeles, Jerusalem, Chapel Hill, New York City, and Berkeley, I met such folks as

Sidney and Emily Kark, Eva and Harry Phillips, Jack Geiger, Art Rubel, and Shirley Lindenbaum, who were gracious in sharing their time, memories, and many published and unpublished books and papers.

In 1988 I moved to the Harvard Institute for International Development, where many of my ideas about interdisciplinary exchanges were tested and revised during seven years of work in 10 countries. I am grateful to Richard Cash, Heidi Clyne, Fitzroy Henry, Bradley Nixon, Jon Simon, and Laura Tesler for providing a stimulating and supportive environment in which to confront new ideas and try to come up with creative solutions to unexpected problems. Johannes Sommerfeld was my intellectual colleague in the social sciences at the Institute. I continue to appreciate and benefit from his persistent enthusiasm for the topic.

In the early 1990s I started sharing my ideas about anthropology and epidemiology with Spanish-language audiences in Latin America. This was made possible primarily through teaching in the International Course on Applied Epidemiology run by Mexico's Ministry of Health and through classes I gave at the Center for the Study of State and Society in Buenos Aires, Argentina; the National Institute of Public Health in Cuernavaca, Mexico; and the Universidad Austral in Valdivia, Chile. I am grateful to these institutions for creating opportunities for me to develop and disseminate many of the ideas expressed here. Mario Bronfman has been a colleague and friend for most of my professional career, and he was instrumental in helping me develop and teach the ideas written in this book through an appointment at Mexico's National Institute of Public Health. Ana Langer, Carlos Coimbra, Jr., Edmundo Granda, Roberto Tapia, Hernan Manzelli, Monica Gogna, Silvina Ramos, and Mariana Romero helped me generously despite their busy schedules. Steve Gehlbach and Harris Pastides at the School of Public Health of the University of Massachusetts and Richard Cash at the School of Public Health at Harvard also helped me learn how to teach this material. Trinity College, through a sabbatical leave and faculty research grant, gave me almost all the time I needed to finish this book.

A number of students have given me research and editorial assistance on this project over the years, including Dorothy Francoeur, Jessica LaPointe, Cynthia Lopez, Andrew Noymer, Brian Page, Camvan Phu, and Elisabeth Woodhams. Librarians at Mount Holyoke College; Trinity College; the Watkinson Library; University of California, Berkeley, School of Public Health; and the Epidemiology Division of Mexico's Ministry of Health all helped find references. Friends and colleagues Beth Conklin, Kitty Corbett, Joe Eisenberg, Mitch Feldman, Craig Janes, Jane Kramer, Lois McCloskey, Steven Katz, Dan Perlman, and Frank Zimmerman helped me to think more synthetically about interdisciplinary work and modeled it themselves. Fernando Barros, Jim Carey, Robert Hahn, and Paul Slovic graciously provided important data and references, and Jennifer Fichera and Luiselle Rivera gave secretarial assistance at critical moments.

Those who read and commented on chapter drafts also made welcome contributions to this work, including Charles Briggs, Mario Bronfman, Peter Guarnaccia, Don Joralemon, Abby Marean, Meredith Miller, Gerry Oppenheimer, Mariana Romero, Jay Schensul, Jeremy Sussman, and Lissy Woodhams, as well as anonymous reviewers. Jessica Kuper originally asked me to write this book, but I owe my largest debt to Alan Harwood, master editor and extraordinarily patient advisor.

Many of the ideas in this book have been traveling with me for a long time. Portions of Chapter 2 are drawn from Trostle (1986a and 1986b) and from Trostle and Sommerfeld (1996). Parts of Chapter 3 were first presented in 1997 at an International Symposium on the Role of Medical Anthropology in Infectious Disease Control at Heidelberg University and in 1999 at the American Anthropological Association annual meeting. Early drafts of Chapter 4 were presented at the Department of Social Medicine at Harvard University in 1990 and at the annual meeting of the American Anthropological Association in 1993. Early versions of Chapter 5 were presented at the 1995 and 1998 meetings of the American Anthropological Association and at the London School of Hygiene and Tropical Medicine in 1999. Portions of Chapter 7 were presented at the joint meeting of the Society for Medical Anthropology and the Society for Applied Anthropology in 2000, the Sixth Latin American Congress of Social Science and Medicine in Peru in 2001, and the CIEPP/COTES meeting in Bolivia in 2001. I am grateful to the audiences at all these venues for their questions and suggestions.

I now fully understand why so many authors dedicate books to their families. My parents, John and Sue Trostle, always encouraged me to be curious and to question boundaries. Noah and Juliana graciously gave up their dad to this book for more time than any of us wanted. And my wife, Lynn Morgan, continues to be my first and last reader. This book is for them.

Epidemiology and Culture

1   Introduction

I used to work on the 19th floor of a building overlooking the Hudson River in upper Manhattan. I was often fascinated by the ever-shifting traffic patterns down below on the busy six-lane Henry Hudson Parkway. A rush-hour accident could bring three lanes of traffic to a halt when a knot of cars backed up behind police cars and ambulances. Unobstructed traffic going the other way would soon jam up, too, as drivers slowed their vehicles and craned their necks to see what had happened. The delays took longer to clear than to form, sometimes persisting an hour or more after an accident had been removed.

This memory of my traffic-observing days came back to me when I thought about how to explain the difference between a "group of individuals" and a "population." I remembered drivers in their vehicles down below, each making decisions about how fast and how close to follow the car in front, looking for a quick exit and trying to catch a glimpse of torn metal or bodies. The sum of the eagerness, frustration, and curiosity of this group of commuters was more than a series of momentary glances or flashes of brake lights. Individual drivers' thoughts and acts, added together over time, turned into traffic delays that themselves *created* additional glances and brake lights and sometimes even new accidents. Individual cars passed through, but their movement created traffic patterns that endured. Drivers and traffic followed related but different rules, and neither was reducible to the other.

I.   Patterns of Disease and Patterns of Culture

Human reactions to disease also create patterns. Imagine a Peruvian fisherman who ate contaminated shellfish in January 1991, contracted cholera, and died. Individuals in his town gathered to wash the body and to mourn the deceased. They drank and ate together, finding companionship. But some of the participants were exposed to cholera in the shared water. Their travels after the funeral changed the likelihood of exposure for many others, and the number of people they saw and the activities they undertook further influenced the spread of the disease. In April 1991, cholera broke out in mountain villages when recently infected but still asymptomatic workers from the coast traveled home to celebrate Easter. Their behavior as a group created patterns that could not be deduced from the sum of their individual actions. Individual decisions and epidemic patterns are partly separable but clearly linked.

Closely related to the kinds of individual decisions and behavioral patterns we have been talking about, culture also influences human health and the patterning of disease. Our total way of life (work, food, activities), combined with our learned behavior (including knowledge, lies, and misunderstandings), our techniques for adjusting to the environment, and our ways of feeling and believing all influence our susceptibility to illness. Some argue that they become written into our genes, and they certainly become written into our bone structure and musculature. Migrant farm workers, for example, have different diseases than coal miners, and Central American men who wield machetes all day for their whole lives often develop one arm longer than the other.

Bodies and pathogens are determined not just by physical actions but by beliefs about what is important. Beliefs are powerful motivators. The disproportionate mortality among infant girls in some South Asian nations is partly an outcome of cultural preferences for sons over daughters (Sen 1992). In cultures where injections are thought to be stronger than pills, a town might have several specialized injectionists on call to administer to the sick (Reeler 2000). And diagnostic preferences among physicians in different countries are responsible for some of the national differences in rates of depression, low blood pressure, and infant mortality (Payer 1988). Rates of morbidity (sickness) and mortality (death) are determined in part by cultural scripts that specify how, where, and when to behave in certain ways.

The influence of culture can be seen in how people care for symptoms before they receive a diagnosis. Groups vary in their willingness to undertake preventive measures; they vary in how they perceive and classify symptoms. Across the world, people employ diverse markers to decide who will be labeled disease-ridden or contagious; they differentially rank which diseases are seen as important or unimportant. What treatment, if any, sick people choose, whether they take medication, how they manipulate their diseases for other ends, whether therapy succeeds – culture influences diseases through these pathways as well as through the patterned work of nerves, muscles, and bones. Whether one thinks of body disorder as influenced by Chinese energy meridians, Tibetan pulses, Latin American hot/cold states, or immune system function is largely a product of where one is and with whom one interacts. Available healing traditions range from the grand and ancient ones of Chinese acupuncture or Greek humoral pathology of blood and bile to more recent precepts of homeopathy or chiropractic in North America. Biomedicine is one particularly widespread form of therapy in the world today, which bases its treatments on a combination of empirical tests and custom. It is a cultural system like the others, often competing with them, less frequently collaborating.

Yet cultural meanings are also local and contested. This aspect of culture highlights its dynamic, changing quality and gives weight to forces of change and interaction. From this perspective, culture is constantly being transformed. People within groups may be aware of group norms, but those norms themselves change over time, and people choose to reject the norms or manipulate their behavior within them. For example, human beauty standards, and their health-related consequences, change dramatically over time. The corset allowed one set of health problems (muscle atrophy, liver damage) to emerge, whereas a century later breast augmentation caused others (pain, scar tissue, implant rupture). Food preferences, time pressure, and large-scale industrial meal production combine to create a new epidemic of obesity based on "fast food" and sedentism.

Cultural categories not only change through time, but they also can be differentially manipulated by people interacting within a web of relationships embedded in a larger material and social context. In that context, individuals pick and choose different aspects of culture to form their own identities; they manipulate cultural symbols, transform them, and combine them in unexpected ways that can protect health or promote disease. Statements about "culture," whether made by local "natives" or well-intentioned "outsiders," need to be evaluated not only in terms of their content but also in terms of the purposes of those who assert them.

This book describes the connections between patterns of disease and patterns of culture to highlight the creative interdisciplinary ways by which researchers are confronting today's vexing and complex health challenges. By creating conversations across disciplines, students and practicing professionals are better able to collaborate across disciplines, design successful health interventions, and communicate more broadly and clearly with both professional and popular audiences (Dunn 1979). These processes will help develop more appropriate health policies, deepen understandings of disease causation and treatment, and create more effective actions to enhance health and prevent disease.

II.   Epidemiology and Medical Anthropology

Both epidemiology and medical anthropology are scientific disciplines that search for patterns of disease and behavior. They both have humanity at their core. The disciplines are separated by history and tradition – epidemiology tends to be statistical and quantitative, anthropology textual and qualitative, but this book brings them together. My vision of an integrated and interdisciplinary dialogue has been created, and is shared, by many like-minded anthropologists and epidemiologists who appreciate the value of collaborating on a common project. (See, for example, Fleck and Ianni 1958, Dunn and Janes 1986, Frankel et al. 1991, Hahn 1995, Inhorn 1995, and Dressler et al. 1997.)

Epidemiology is derived from the Greek *epi* meaning "upon," *demos* meaning "the populace or common people," and *logos* meaning "word." Epidemiology is literally the study of what is upon the populace, referring specifically to the burden of disease. Because epidemics were once the most obviously burdensome of diseases, the two words overlap. But epidemiology is more than the study of epidemics. It is more conventionally defined as the study of the distribution and determinants of disease in human populations. Members of this discipline produce descriptions of health and disease patterns and trends rather than laboratory experiments or case reports. They focus on populations using statistics and probabilities.

A significant part of the practice of epidemiology consists of trying to separate out the patterns of disease and exposure from patterns caused by data collection methods. Epidemiologic data can be subject to systematic error from influences such as fallible memory or faulty record-keeping. Such data also can systematically differ from true values based on age or sex of interviewer, sensitivity of behavior, or time since event. Epidemiologists try to minimize the likelihood that they will confuse patterns of systematic error with patterns generated from the health-related effects of age, diet, wealth, exercise, occupation, or other so-called risk factors that get such attention in the press.

Epidemiologists describe disease patterns using data about the past or data collected from the present into the future. They use *prospective* study designs to follow a group of people over time, tracking their exposure to potential causes of disease and observing whether rates of disease differ according to whether or not a person was exposed. For example, a study might track oral contraceptive use in a group of nurses over 15 years and conclude that their likelihood of getting breast cancer was influenced by whether they took birth control pills. *Retrospective* studies look at records or reports of people who already have a disease, comparing the proportion of people who do not have a prior history of a particular behavior or exposure with the proportion of those who do. For example, researchers might begin with a group of adults with lung cancer and compare the proportion of smokers and nonsmokers. Epidemiologists make these types of comparisons to investigate the factors that increase (or reduce) people's probability of acquiring a disease.

When epidemiologists work across different countries and within diverse groups in a single country they come inevitably into contact with cultural difference. It is tempting to think that culture[1] can serve as a new explanatory variable, capable of predicting and explaining significant portions of observed variation in behavior and disease. That culture matters but should not be treated as a single variable is an important premise of this volume.

I argue throughout this book that epidemiologists should devote the same attention to culture that they have given to "social" factors over the past few decades. Social epidemiology is the branch of epidemiology that most directly attends to the health-related effects of social organization, and in many ways it most closely approximates the goals I outline in this book. Social epidemiologists look at the health effects of income, wealth, job stress, class, social support, inequality, and occupation. They define societies as groups of people who interact in specific ways, live in specifiable places, and share some common set of values. My treatment of "culture" parallels how epidemiologists use the word "society." But it leads to closer scrutiny of the unexamined assumptions behind epidemiologic variables and measurements, takes more account of international variability, and attends more often to the influence of categories and perceptions.

The concept of a *cultural epidemiology* focused on the health-related effects of behavior and belief also merits attention. This book emphasizes culture more than society because I want to argue for a complementary alternative to social epidemiology, one that focuses attention on disease classification, meaning, risk, and behavior in addition to social variables such as income, marital status, and occupation. Culture is less widely appreciated in the epidemiological worldview, but it has explanatory power and effectiveness comparable to the concept of society. Culture can be a slippery concept; it both contains and describes many meanings. For

---

[1] The concept of *culture* has a long history, and the word itself has a long list of definitions. The anthropologist Clyde Kluckhohn (1949) provides several competing definitions, including "the total way of life of a people," "learned behavior," "a set of techniques for adjusting both to the external environment and to other people," and "a way of thinking, feeling, and believing." Clifford Geertz has defined culture as a set of symbols that are organized into systems of meaning. He wrote, "Believing, with Max Weber, that man is an animal suspended in webs of significance he himself has spun, I take culture to be those webs, and the analysis of it to be therefore not an experimental science in search of law but an interpretive one in search of meaning" (1973:5). One can distinguish between culture as a set of patterns *for* behavior and the patterns *of* behavior that emerge from a group following a set of cultural rules over time, akin to the traffic patterns I describe at the beginning of this chapter.

research or policy purposes it is sometimes better unpacked and transformed into smaller, better-defined, operational categories. It is nevertheless useful as an orienting framework, and this book will show how this can be done and why it matters.

Like epidemiologists, medical anthropologists also search for patterns, but they find them in culturally patterned responses to disease. Medical anthropologists study the afflictions facing humankind and how human groups organize themselves to treat and explain the causes of suffering. They analyze the understanding and interpretation of healing, illness, and health, as well as the environmental, biological, behavioral, and cultural determinants of disease. To do so, they use a variety of methods, including long- and short-term fieldwork, structured observations, open-ended interviews, and a variety of survey and group interview techniques.

Both epidemiology and medical anthropology have domestic and international applications. Traditionally, epidemiologists tended to study problems within their national borders, whereas medical anthropologists tended to study foreign cultures. But diseases rarely respect human borders, and human beings often cross them. As epidemiologists increasingly examine patterns of diseases across borders, and as medical anthropologists increasingly look at cultural diversity within borders, their geographic scopes have converged. This book therefore will refer to a broad range of studies undertaken both within the United States and worldwide (and see Coimbra and Trostle 2004 for related work about Latin America).

Neither anthropology nor epidemiology is a monolithic discipline. Each comprises multiple theoretical orientations using a varied but limited set of common research methods. Some medical anthropologists emphasize the interpretation of suffering; others assess physical and social adaptations to high altitude. Some epidemiologists study disease strains in a single town, others the movement of diseases across the globe. Thus some themes within each discipline may lend themselves more readily to collaboration.

Although my accent in this book is on collaboration between the disciplines, I also emphasize the unique and separate contributions of each one. I do this for three reasons: first, the history and nature of interdisciplinary collaboration between anthropology and epidemiology are still relatively unexplored. It is therefore important to highlight what methods and theories each discipline has contributed to prior joint studies. Second, when interdisciplinary collaboration is effective but still marginal, a focus on disciplines makes it easier to explore the separate contributions of each side toward helping or hindering that collaboration. Third, I argue that even though medical anthropology and epidemiology do have many "joint ventures," training programs and research incentives do not yet push the fields together as often as they could and should. In the absence of a long interdisciplinary tradition, I hope that my examples and claims for the relevance of one discipline might spark enthusiasm among adherents of the other.

For example, from an anthropological perspective, epidemiology is one particular system of knowledge production; it is, in short, a culture. By analyzing the categories and assumptions of epidemiologists, anthropologists see that epidemiologists work within a system of rules and expectations just as do acupuncturists, chiropractors, or shamans. Anthropologists use the term "reflexivity" to refer to their efforts to understand their own assumptions, biases, and conventions. But without the benefit of cross-cultural comparison or a tradition of reflexivity, epidemiologists might find it harder to see cultural influences in their own work. Most of their studies are done in and for their own familiar cultures, are based in biomedical theories of illness causation, and are justified within a particular research framework that celebrates empirical tests and falsifiable hypotheses. For these reasons, epidemiologists are likely to describe the rules of their research as dictated by the scientific method not by cultural rules about professional identity, the qualities of a good measurement, or the effect of politics in science.

One way to notice that epidemiologists are embedded in culture is to think about what influences their measures of disease. Statistical tests, research designs, risk factor definitions, and disease definitions all rise and fall in popularity, and their use is not governed solely by "objective" assessments of their appropriateness for a given question. For example, clinical journals have published multiple and competing recommendations about what kinds of statistical tests should be presented (Sterne and Davey Smith 2001). Computer-based statistical packages and geographic information systems make complex tests and visual representations of quantitative data available to many scientists, when formerly they were available only to a few. Cheap digital storage on computers facilitates collecting and linking massive quantities of patient information, and privacy laws sometimes help and sometimes hinder the use of that information. The categories used to define and thereby "see" human groups vary over time, as shown by the change over the past three decades in U.S. census categories from Black/White/other to self-identified multiethnic categories (U.S. Bureau of the Census 2001a). And the proportion of important clinical studies that involve epidemiologic research varies dramatically from country to country (Takahashi et al. 2001), evidence that the discipline's power and prominence is not everywhere the same.

III.   Applying an Integrated Cultural-Epidemiological Approach

Culture influences the patterning of disease through many pathways, ranging from who is counted to what is noticed to where people obtain help for suffering. Its influence can be seen in the varying ways parents try to protect their children from the common cold, as well as in the differential power of epidemiology across nations. More complete understanding of the range of cultural influences on disease patterning will come as more frequent and profound interactions take place between the disciplines of medical anthropology and epidemiology, among others. Some examples of existing collaborative projects are summarized in this volume. As a start, let us consider a cultural approach to a biomedically accepted entity, epilepsy, and an epidemiological approach to a "culture-specific syndrome," *ataque de nervios*.

People's understandings about disease and therapy influence disease patterns in ways that epidemiologists may not always appreciate. Two very basic concepts in epidemiology, the description of human disease in terms of *incidence* and *prevalence*, can be used to illustrate this suggestion. *Incidence* is the number of people developing a disease over a particular period of time; an incidence rate compares the number of new cases of disease within a defined time period with the total number of susceptible people in a defined population. Incidence matters because it measures the rate of disease change in a population. If epidemiologists want to know how rapidly a disease is developing or disappearing, or to figure out why new cases are appearing, they need to know the incidence of the disease and investigate incident cases. Incidence can be thought of as measuring the force or pressure of disease: it describes how quickly disease moves through populations.

Prevalence, on the other hand, is the number of people having a disease at a particular point in time, and a prevalence rate compares the number of existing cases with the total population. Prevalence can be thought of as measuring the weight, rather than the force, of disease. Prevalence matters because it measures the burden of disease on a population. If epidemiologists want to plan treatment programs or measure the needs of people with a disease in some defined place (no matter whether they have had the disease for a long or a short time), then they need to know the prevalence of the disease.

Prevalence is partly influenced by disease duration. If a disease lasts a long time in an individual, such as diabetes or asthma, the prevalence of that disease in the population will usually be larger than its incidence because more people in the population have the disease at one point in time than develop the disease over a period of time. If a disease like chickenpox or an acute respiratory infection lasts a short time in an individual, incidence in a population will often be larger than prevalence because many people can get the disease over time but fewer will have it at any particular point in time.

A.   A Cultural Epidemiological Study of Epilepsy

In the nineteenth century, Oliver Wendell Holmes, Sr., Professor of Anatomy at Harvard, said, "If I wished to show a student the difficulties of getting at the truth from medical experience, I would give him the history of epilepsy to read" (Holmes 1860). The same could be said of AIDS or of sickle cell trait today, but even 150 years ago epilepsy had a long, convoluted, and contradictory history. The medical historian Owsei Temkin's book, *The Falling Sickness* (1971), recounts how epilepsy has been seen variously over time as a disease caused by spirits, demons, gods, nature, and human will, although physicians now speak quite confidently about this syndrome that they know, measure, diagnose, and treat. The cultural meanings of epilepsy have affected whether and how it becomes visible to epidemiologists and what this means for estimates of its incidence, prevalence, causes, and outcomes.

Epilepsy is the most common serious condition seen by neurologists. It is estimated to have an annual incidence of about 50 per 100,000 in industrialized countries and a prevalence of about 5 to 6 per 1,000 (Hauser and Kurland 1975). The lifetime risk of any individual having a seizure is about 5%. For physicians, epilepsy is a brain disorder characterized by recurrent seizures caused by abnormal electrical activity (uncoordinated electrical discharges) in the brain. From a clinical point of view, epilepsy is the name for a group of disorders characterized by recurrent seizures, which can manifest as jerking motions of particular limbs, sensations and thoughts, or convulsions of the whole body.

Neurologists think of epilepsy as having two components: the seizures themselves and their underlying cause. They can treat the seizures with anticonvulsant medication, but they can rarely explain why seizures develop in the first place. When a patient asks, "Why me?," the doctor often does not know. Nor can a doctor specify when the seizures might stop. Physicians label epilepsy a chronic disease, yet patients experience seizures as sporadic and (usually) unpredictable events. They wonder how long they must be seizure-free to be considered epilepsy-free, and they wonder how they will know whether they are seizure-free while they remain on anticonvulsant medication. This combination of factors – uncertainties about the cause, the prognosis, and the end point – encourages people with epilepsy to develop their own explanations for the condition and to adjust their medications accordingly.

So how can the concept of culture help us understand incidence and prevalence? A cultural-epidemiological approach shows that local meanings and management strategies for this disease influence the number and severity of cases that come to the attention of epidemiologists and thus help to determine whose disease gets counted and how disabling the disease looks. It employs both of the meanings of culture introduced earlier in this chapter: a set of beliefs and practices learned and transmitted through time, and a set of contingent processes subject to manipulation and change. Through the prism of epilepsy, and of seizures more generally, we can see how symptoms and prognosis, personal and social reactions, and categorization and measurement all help to create patterns of disease in populations.

Olmsted County, Minnesota, has been the site of an important epidemiologic study of epilepsy in the community since the mid-1950s. Almost all residents of Olmsted County receive their health care from the Mayo Clinic in Rochester, Minnesota, and other health facilities in the county also make their records available for study by Mayo personnel. When I worked at Mayo in 1985 I studied the medical records of 199 county residents aged 18 to 59 who received care for epilepsy. I interviewed 127 adults from this group who had active epilepsy (defined as having had a seizure or taken anticonvulsants within five years prior to January 1, 1980). My objective was to understand the differences between physician and patient perspectives on epilepsy, its impact, and its care.

Interviewees were asked a series of closed and open-ended questions about how they managed their condition, what they thought had caused it, what others thought of it, and what differences it had made in their lives. Some of the respondents used biomedical language to describe their condition, labeling their seizures as grand or petit mal and talking about seeing the results of brain scans or brain waves. But they also used a large variety of nonmedical terms to describe their seizures, including fainting or dizzy spells, zonking out, passing out, sleeping spells, blackouts, popping off, and jumps. Some attributed seizures to stress, diet, or emotional pressure, even when physicians were unable to confirm such connections. Seventy-nine percent of 127 people mentioned classical biomedical categories (illness, trauma, physiologic problems) as the ultimate cause of their seizures (i.e., why they were susceptible to having seizures), even though physicians identified causes in only 14% (Trostle 1987:24–28). When explaining what triggered particular seizures, these respondents resorted primarily to categories of stress or emotions (55% of respondents), sleep deprivation (26%), or tiredness (21%).

The following quotes illustrate a few of the ways residents of Rochester described their epilepsy. Esther was a middle-aged married housewife, a high school graduate who used to be an office manager. Her seizures started in high school, and she stopped taking anticonvulsant medication after 5 years without a seizure. Her seizures started again about 10 years after she stopped taking anticonvulsant medication:

I just have a problem. I don't know why. They still haven't said, 'You're an epileptic.' They say, 'Because you've had it this many years you must have a seizure disorder, but we don't know what it is.' But it's still abnormal – if you fall and break your leg, that's normal – this isn't.

George was a 19-year-old drug store clerk with one year of college who was now living at home. His seizures began when he was 8 and continued until he was 16. He said he thought his seizures started originally because of some "insufficiency in my system." He wasn't quite sure whether they were seizures or not. He said his mother urged him to call his seizures "sleeping spells":

My doctor says these are seizures – something not controlled from me, but from body chemistry. But my social worker says these are anxiety attacks. I think that means I cause them myself – they're my fault. Right now I think they *are* anxiety attacks, but my doctor... Most people think that their doctor is God, so I guess since he said they're seizures, they're seizures. So... whatever he says, goes. But I just wonder if they are anxiety attacks. Like wondering why I'd think I'd not had one in a while, then have one later, just a few hours after thinking about it.

These passages highlight the distance between what people know from their doctors about their epilepsy and what they would like to know about their epilepsy. Esther is concerned about the absence of a label for her condition and about whether to call it a "normal" disease. George wants to find who or what is responsible for his seizures. He struggles between his doctor's offer of chemistry as culprit and his social worker's implicit suggestion that seizures are brought on by his own anxiety.

Studies I later did in Ecuador and Kenya among people with epileptic seizures showed they had quite different interpretations of their illness. People in the highland north of Ecuador often mentioned pent-up rage, frustration, suffering, and "nerves" as causes of particular seizures, while they used heredity to explain why one was exposed to the possibility of having seizures in the first place. In Kenya, physical causes such as malaria, bad blood, and trauma were mentioned as causes of seizures by people in the Rift Valley, as were cognitive processes such as thinking about problems or imagining things. Some in Kenya thought epilepsy was contagious, particularly if one touched a person with epilepsy during the seizure. Consequently, in rural areas where people cooked over open fires, some people were not moved away from fires during their seizures. Fully one-third of the 89 people I interviewed in Kenya bore large keloid scars from such burns, further stigmatizing them. Some thought epilepsy was a form of supernatural punishment for their misdeeds. Strikingly, few people with epilepsy in Kenya identified epilepsy as something involving the brain: 71% of interviewees said their seizures were originally caused by malaria, 13% said they were caused by pneumonia, and only 13% called it epilepsy.

The narratives of people from Ecuador and Kenya reflect quite different strategies of understanding where their seizures came from and how they should be managed from those of the Minnesotans. One striking difference in these strategies is the use of both biomedical and nonbiomedical types of health resources, as well as recourse to (or explicit rejection of) supernatural explanations of seizure causation. This is how Isabel, a middle-aged woman from a small town in highland Ecuador, explained the origin of her seizures and how she took care of them:

Well, it must be about three years ago, three years it must be, when I had it the first time. The first time I had an "attack" (*ataque*) was late one Sunday afternoon. I was here alone, and then my brother and his wife took me right away to the hospital, where I spent eight days. They took good care of me there, but I can't tell you what medication I took because I don't remember. They gave me pills, injections, and an intravenous solution. They said . . . The Doctor said it was from all the nervousness that I had and that's what caused this to happen. After three months I went back. They gave me some more injections, no pills. They told me not to be so nervous. When I get nervous I should go do something else, take a walk or go to a party.

About six months later I had another one. Then I went back to the hospital, and they gave me these pills. I took them every once in a while, when I felt quite nervous, or when I thought I would lose consciousness. I took a pill with water from *malva olorosa*, a plant which grows around here which is really good for nerves.

I never thought this came from *mal hecho* [sorcery] because if it had, it would have continued to be bad. I wouldn't have been able to cure it with the medicine I took. Look, I came to have this problem with my nerves because I was living mostly by myself, so I worried a lot about the same things over and over again. My husband had a business. He went to work elsewhere, and sometimes he said he'd come home and he didn't, so I worried. The people around here are different; they're not so good now. You might say they're troublemakers. They try to rob you, so I started to think maybe they hit my husband, maybe he got assaulted.

Maybe that's why he didn't come home yet. So that's why these started: little by little, this is what caused these attacks. It's not that someone hexed me.

Mary, a mother of a 10-year-old boy with seizures who lived in a medium-sized town in Kenya, used different words to describe her ideas about epilepsy and how she sought treatment for him. Note her mention of a broad variety of health resources quite different from those mentioned in the Ecuadorian case. Also note the complex consultations with multiple practitioners when cures did not work as promised, as well as the perceived need to hide use of local traditional healers for fear of being accused of practicing witchcraft.

This illness was first caused by malaria and pneumonia. When he first got this illness, we rushed him to the hospital. After we visited the hospital, our relatives told us to go and see a *mganga* [curer]. They said he inherited the illness. Some friends tell us to take the child to the curer, while others tell us to take him to Kenyatta Hospital, where we will get doctors who know what the illness is. We decided to go to a *mganga* because at Kenyatta Hospital one can't just be treated unless you know somebody.

We took the child to three doctors. The last place discharged him when he felt a little bit better. They said he was cured. But he wasn't.

We went to three traditional healers to cure him. The first one said the child had inherited the illness. He told us to take a chicken and a goat's head to him. We did. He slaughtered the chicken the same day before we left. I don't know whether he ate it or not. The second healer told us the child had inherited the illness. He asked for a chicken and a bird called *chaluu* so that he could exchange the illness with those things. The boy's father decided not to take the things because the illness was persisting even after visiting the first healer, and he was already tired of their treatment.

The third healer asked for a red chicken and a goat. We took the chicken but not the goat. He looked at it and said that the toes of the chicken should be removed and tied to the child for three days. We could tie the chicken nails on at night and take them off in the morning. We feared our son would be seen with such stuff when at school, and people might charge us with practicing witchcraft. This didn't work, either.

In Minnesota, respondents with epilepsy tended to explain the causes of their condition using biomedical language, even when their own physicians would not or could not. In Ecuador, an emotional idiom was used, referring to nerves, and the dangers of fear, anger, and frustration. In Kenya, epilepsy was sufficiently stigmatized that people with the diagnosis labeled it as a manifestation of malaria instead. Seizures demand an explanation, and explanations lead to a series of help-seeking and treatment strategies. Local culture provides the interpretive frameworks, which the anthropologist classifies as biological, personal, or supernatural, without making judgments as to whether they are plausible or "true" according to biomedical standards. Two of the causal categories recognized by people with epilepsy – emotional stress and supernatural interference – are not commonly recognized in biomedicine as causes of disease. When sufferers attribute causes to nervousness or the supernatural, they often resort to nonbiomedical healing traditions, or they mix biomedicine with other traditions. They may take anticonvulsant pills with stress-reducing teas as Isabel did or combine hospital visits with treatments by indigenous curers as Mary did. And they watch carefully to see what seems to work.

In the United States and elsewhere, patients suffer from the label "epilepsy," as well as the disease. Because ongoing use of medications for epilepsy is part of the medical definition of a "case" of epilepsy, patients face incentives to stop taking their medications to see if they will have a seizure. Also, the diagnostic label hinders daily life because most forms of insurance are more expensive for people with epilepsy, and a driver's license is sometimes impossible to retain. People therefore feel pressured to rid themselves of the diagnosis as soon as possible. This is one reason George's mother urged him to label his seizures sleeping spells instead.

Physicians (and especially neurologists) also have a stake in the definition of epilepsy. They help to determine its incidence and prevalence because they decide whether and when to apply the diagnosis of "epilepsy," and they are responsible for deciding when a patient should no longer be considered "an epileptic." But in some respects they serve the government in a set of surveillance and assessment functions that extend beyond counting for public health purposes. For example, they establish the severity of a case and whether it poses limits to safe driving or work capacity. They also help to determine eligibility for government disability payments. Because the treatment for epilepsy has specific and sometimes deleterious side effects, physicians determine who must continue to be treated and for how long. There is a complex social negotiation between doctor and patient, and a patient's interest in avoiding or limiting the diagnosis of epilepsy may complicate the physician's task.

Epilepsy also poses a challenge to epidemiologists eager to group cases and explore their common features. Epidemiologists of epilepsy focus on three defining characteristics: presence of more than one seizure, timing of the most recent seizure (within the past five years), and behavior (patient still taking anticonvulsant medications). But these criteria are far from ideal. They require accurate surveillance and reporting, and they are influenced by individual patient desires to eliminate the disease label by stopping the medication or by underreporting seizure activity. Some of the miscommunication may be intentional, but epilepsy is also a neurological problem that can affect cognition and memory. Can respondents clearly describe their past seizures? Can they recall past exposure to potential causes of epilepsy? The physiology and experience of this condition influence how it is reported and by whom, and this also helps determine measures of its incidence and prevalence.

People with epilepsy do not necessarily even *want* to be visible in the general population (Beran et al. 1985). This has implications for epidemiologists who want to know what functional limitations the condition may cause because there may be systematic differences in intellectual ability and level of handicap between those who can hide their condition and those who cannot. For this reason, epilepsy may look particularly disabling among those attending specialty clinics and more benign among people with epilepsy in the general population, who may not be receiving specialty care. This is another area where epidemiologic results can be influenced by patterns of service use.

By combined anthropological and epidemiological approaches, my study in Rochester, Minnesota, showed that published reports from specialized treatment clinics overestimated the social damage created by epilepsy compared with studies conducted among the general population (Trostle 1987). Before this study, almost all published reports of the outcomes of epilepsy came from sources able to marshal relatively large numbers of cases, primarily specialty clinic populations or members of service-based groups such as the Epilepsy Foundation of America or self-help groups. These groups could be expected to show more severe problems than community-based samples because they include more people who have current management problems, are more severely afflicted, or are less able to cope with their illness. Indeed, Figure 1.1 shows that my pure community-based sample in Rochester had the lowest frequency of problems; mixed self-help and clinic groups had the middle level; and a pure clinic-based sample had the most problems.

Does this mean that prior research wrongly described the types of problems associated with epilepsy? It may have overstated the frequency of such problems among all people with epilepsy by assuming that cases drawn from specialty care centers represent those in the community at large – this is the essence of what epidemiologists call selection bias. But in fact the problem of generalizing from clinic to community cuts both ways. It can underestimate as well as overestimate problems: if groups like urban minorities are less likely to seek medical care for seizures, then they may be even more negatively affected by epilepsy than clinic-based studies would suggest. This is why it is necessary to pay attention to the social location of cases, to specify more completely the variable effects of epilepsy among different groups.

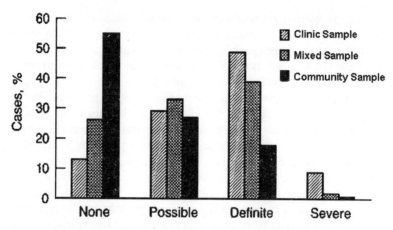

Figure 1.1. Comparison of percentages of subjects in three samples (clinic, mixed community and clinic, and pure community) with problem scores in four regions of elevation on a Psychosocial Functioning Scale of the Washington Psychosocial Seizure Inventory. *Source*: Trostle et al. 1989:635. Copyright by Lippincott, Williams & Wilkins, 1989.

From the point of view of epidemiology, epilepsy offers a lesson for how measurement tools themselves can raise the status of some medical conditions and ignore others. Epilepsy was relatively unimportant on the worldwide disease priority list when diseases were ranked according to their contribution to infant or child mortality because it rarely kills. Epilepsy also was neglected because its symptoms resemble some stigmatized types of mental illness. The condition began to get increased research attention and funding following development of new ranking systems for diseases, particularly the Disability-Adjusted Life Year, or DALY, developed by the World Bank in 1993. Because the DALY measured the disabling potential of diseases in addition to their mortality and duration, epilepsy jumped to prominence. The World Bank labeled it as one of the 10 most important diseases among all children 5 to 14 years of age in developing countries (World Bank 1993). It exacted its toll through school withdrawal, social isolation, and inability to find work. The DALY method of categorizing disease allowed the detrimental effects of epilepsy to become more visible, thus increasing the research attention and health service funding directed at this condition.

Epilepsy is noninfectious and chronic; it disables both young and old. It poses a number of challenges to epidemiologists who would study its incidence and prevalence or public health practitioners who seek to prevent it. Because it is defined largely by its symptoms (seizures), diagnosis depends largely on patient or observer report. Because its symptoms are episodic or even rare, it resists those trying to define duration or the onset of new events. Epilepsy illustrates how individual and household management of disease channels people into different healing systems, where varied diagnoses and therapies are offered. Its culture-specific interpretations illustrate the discrepancies between lay and professional explanations of cause, course, and consequence.

In summary, the incidence and prevalence of epilepsy are influenced by many forces, some natural and some social and cultural. Its symptoms prompt specific reactions (e.g., social isolation) and explanations (e.g., biochemical imbalance, supernatural force) that vary from place to place even when the symptoms do not. And these reactions and explanations in turn influence other aspects of the epidemiology of the condition – its association in rural Kenya with keloid scars from burns from kitchen fires, for example, or its disabling potential, and even people's willingness to acknowledge its existence. People's reactions to disease can influence epidemiology because epidemiology is primarily an observational science that relies on people's reports. (This issue will be further discussed in Chapter 4.)

B.   *A Cultural-Epidemiological Study of* Ataques de Nervios

Imagine Rosa, a middle-aged woman from Puerto Rico who moved with her family to New York City in 1953. This was toward the beginning of a major shift of population from Puerto Rico to the mainland United States, one that in a single decade would turn New York City into what some called the largest city in Puerto Rico. Rosa cared deeply for her children, and when her oldest son died in a traffic accident in 1958 she was inconsolable. Her crying became more intense at the funeral, and on her departure from the building she collapsed to the ground, unconscious and shaking.

Had this happened at her former home in Puerto Rico, her relatives would probably have known she was having a nervous attack, or *ataque de nervios*, prompted by extreme grief. Such *ataques* were an acceptable cultural response to strong emotions like grief and anger. There people would have known Rosa needed her family to rally around her, and they would perhaps have taken her to a local *espiritista* (spirit medium) for a spiritual cleansing that would help heal her grief. But in New York City the funeral home director thought she was having some kind of epileptic seizure and called an ambulance.

Rosa was taken to the emergency room, where physicians found she had none of the signs of an epileptic seizure. They suspected this to be some sort of mental breakdown, and they referred Rosa to a psychiatrist. But Rosa and her family were offended that the hospital staff thought she was crazy, and they refused to return to the hospital. By now physicians had seen many of these types of seizures among Puerto Ricans, so many that a psychiatrist wrote an article in 1961 titled, "The Puerto Rican Syndrome" (Fernández-Marina 1961). The thesis of this and similar articles published around that time was that Puerto Ricans were particularly unsophisticated at managing their emotions and were somehow culturally predisposed to having these kinds of "hysterical" displays. But this reaction revealed more about clinicians' lack of cultural knowledge about Puerto Ricans than it did about mental and emotional processes among Puerto Ricans. An *ataque* accepted in one land became a syndrome denigrated in another (Harwood 1977). This translation involved the movement of Puerto Rican people into new places and their transformation from a dominant group into a minority group.

Seizures are a dramatic instance of loss of bodily control, and they often prompt some kind of social response. But not all dramatic body movements are epileptic, the product of uncontrolled storms of neurons firing in the brain. Trance states, fainting spells, trembling limbs, and facial contortions are all socially recognized ways to manifest a variety of types of acute distress. A large variety of such non-epileptic seizure categories have been identified in the United States, ranging from what is called "jumping Frenchman" in Maine to "falling out" in Georgia and Florida to "moth madness" in Arizona. The *ataques de nervios* in Puerto Rico also have been described in the Dominican Republic and elsewhere in Latin America, and many other "shaking syndromes" exist elsewhere.

These categories do not correspond to any neurological diagnosis; rather they are examples of what have been called "idioms of distress" or "culture-bound syndromes." Labels like these acknowledge that some forms of distress do not match any existing biomedical diagnoses yet form a coherent set of symptoms that are consistent across sites.

How does one study the causes and prevalence and consequences of such indicators of human distress when they cannot be traced to an electroencephalogram reading or brain tumor and have labels not developed by physicians? For much of the 1960s descriptions of *ataques* came from emergency room patients, and they were thought to be a problem limited primarily to Puerto Rican patients. But in the 1970s anthropologists with an interest in medicine and psychology began to look at *nervios* in other sites and discovered that these types of physical responses to stress had many names and existed in many places (Low 1985, Weidman 1979). A study in Miami in the early 1970s looked at eight months of reports of instances where emergency services were requested. A team of scientists

removed all instances of epilepsy, trauma, fainting, heart trouble, diabetes, alcohol use, and the like and found that about 12% of the 3700 case
reports might have been the kinds of seizures, semi-conscious, and unconscious states described as *ataques* or as falling out (Lefley 1979). This
study found cases of falling out to be more prevalent in the Black population than in the Latino or Anglo population, and most common among
Latinas and male Blacks and Whites. But all these estimates were tem-
pered by the fact that the researchers had little detail about exactly what
caused the request for emergency services, and they had to wonder
whether their figures might have been influenced by the likelihood with
which different groups (classified by age, gender, skin color, ethnicity, or
physical condition) would call for emergency services in the first place
rather than calling a private physician or doing nothing.

More complex and valid designs were used to study *ataques* in Puerto
Rico and in Mexico in the 1990s. In Puerto Rico, as a result of collaboration between anthropologists, epidemiologists, and psychiatrists, a survey
of psychological symptoms was given to a large population after a series of
damaging storms in the mid-1980s. The survey asked specifically about
ataques de nervios among other symptoms, and it found that about 16%
of respondents reported having had one (Guarnaccia et al. 1993). They
were more common among middle-aged women who had not finished
high school but who had formerly been married. Since the survey design
allowed people who reported having *ataques* to be compared with people
who had not, Guarnaccia and colleagues were able to compare rates of
psychiatric diagnoses between the two groups. They found that people
who reported *ataques* were far more likely to be depressed, anxious, and
suicidal than those who had not. In sum, *ataques* in Puerto Rico did not
overlap exclusively with any single psychiatric disorder. They seem to
be both a way to describe a set of symptoms that occur to people who
are severely anxious or depressed and a way to explain and to promote
particular kinds of reactions to stressful family events.

A similar study of the prevalence and causes of *nervios* was undertaken
in Mexico (Salgado de Snyder et al. 2000). Random sampling of rural
populations was done in two regions, and respondents were asked if they
had ever had *nervios*. About 16% of this sample also responded posi-
tively, with *nervios* again more common among women than men. The
authors concluded that *nervios* in Mexico do not overlap with any existing biomedical category. Rather they are part of a "deteriorating process"
that weakens both body and mind, constituting a "cry for help" that may
lead to more serious mental and physical dysfunction (2000:467).

In summary, collaborative projects between anthropologists, epidemiologists, and others interested in the frequency and causes of mental

disorders have shown that epidemiological tools and concepts can also be applied to forms of disease that do not match well with biomedical categories and diagnoses. Some have called for programs of research that would link anthropology, epidemiology, and clinical research to study culture-bound syndromes such as *nervios* (Guarnaccia and Rogler 1999). This is a positive step, for it suggests that the accumulating evidence about the level and type of illness and distress in a population is not based solely on cases of patients who come to seek medical treatment or cases that easily fit established biomedical categories. These are steps toward measuring the burden of disease as perceived by the population in addition to that perceived by medical professionals. (This issue is discussed in more detail in Chapter 7.)

As with epilepsy, the label of *nervios* helps to determine where people get treated and whether they get counted in standard epidemiologic studies. The physical symptom called a seizure is prompted by a broad variety of both physical and mental causes and is treated by a broad variety of health practitioners. Epidemiologic methods can be used to study the incidence and prevalence of many types of seizures and when combined with anthropological and sociological methods can yield more complex, satisfying, and culturally sensitive explanations of cause and cure.

FOR FURTHER READING

Berkman L. F. and I. Kawachi, eds. 2000. *Social Epidemiology*. New York: Oxford University Press.

Fadiman A. 1996. *The Spirit Catches You and You Fall Down*. New York: Farrar Straus and Giroux.

Gordis L. 2000. *Epidemiology*. 2nd edition. Philadelphia: Saunders.

Hahn R. A. 1995. *Sickness and Healing: An Anthropological Perspective*. New Haven: Yale University Press.

Janes C. R., R. Stall, and S. Gifford, eds. 1986. *Anthropology and Epidemiology*. Dordrecht: Reidel.

Stolley P. D. and T. Lasky. 1995. *Investigating Disease Patterns: The Science of Epidemiology*. New York: Scientific American Library.

Young T. K. 1998. *Population Health: Concepts and Methods*. Oxford: Oxford University Press.

2 The Origins of an Integrated Approach in Anthropology and Epidemiology

Medical anthropology and epidemiology began from a common objective, namely to explain the health of human populations using observational techniques. But with a few notable exceptions, medical anthropologists and epidemiologists rarely had much to do with one another until the last quarter of the twentieth century.

Epidemiologists interested in history commonly trace the origins of their discipline back 2400 years to Hippocratic texts, particularly, *Airs, Waters, Places,* which emphasized environmental factors (seasons, winds, water, position, and soil) in disease causation. But Hippocrates also discussed diseases as attributes of populations, and he emphasized the etiologic significance of the "mode of life" of a town's populace: "whether they are heavy drinkers, taking lunch, and inactive; or athletic, industrious, eating much and drinking little" (Hippocrates 1957:73). Thus an interest in what today might be called "behavioral" or "social" causes of disease predates the terms themselves and certainly comes long before the scientific disciplines organized to investigate them.

Today we divide such health-related knowledge into such fields as medical anthropology, social epidemiology, medical sociology, bioinformatics, and psychoneuroimmunology. Such labeling seems both inevitable and natural – it is hard to think about how else we might categorize our knowledge. But of course, the boundaries between disciplines are not sacrosanct. Integrating knowledge across disciplines involves both communicating ideas across them and recognizing, respecting, and using ideas from multiple disciplines. As we shall see in recounting the history of early anthropological and epidemiological collaborations, interdisciplinary exchanges are most productive when researchers work together to define their questions, objectives, designs, methods, and analyses. Disciplines often impede such collaboration when they proclaim themselves to be the sole owners and only legitimate investigators of particular domains of research and knowledge. In addition, the specialized journals, technical language, and accepted techniques that facilitate communication within each discipline also impede communication outside it. Moreover, the forces that allow some disciplines to capture resources and power prevent other disciplines from entering into interdisciplinary collaboration as equals. Yet attention to common questions and problems, as we shall see, promotes the integration of approaches.

I.   Scientific Attention to the Social Environment in the Nineteenth Century

The origins of exchanges between anthropologists and epidemiologists go back at least to the mid-nineteenth century (Trostle 1986a). Both disciplines were founded at about that time and developed in an environment characterized by rapid social change with dramatic consequences for human health. Factory production fostered urban migration and hazardous working conditions, while scientists and social activists, attuned to the upheaval, examined the impact of these changes on human health.

In parallel, a broad set of theoretical, technological, and bureaucratic developments during the nineteenth century helped to create a focus on disease in populations. In the eighteenth century the medical research had shifted from an emphasis on bodily humors such as blood and bile to a concern with bodily structures such as hearts and skin; only then did health-related research come to focus on specific diseases (Shryock 1961:94). Accurate quantitative descriptions of specific diseases could occur only after they could be identified with a level of certainty and consistency (Susser 1973); thus epidemiologic measurements such as incidence or prevalence were also contingent on the quality of disease diagnosis.

In the eighteenth century hospitals also changed from places of lodging to places to treat the sick. This was critical to accurate diagnosis because it allowed sophisticated procedures to be developed. Physicians working in hospitals began to see for the first time beyond the particularities of their own practices; they could examine many patients with the same disease, be it rare or epidemic. Consistent and general diagnostic portraits of a disease thus could be built out of many individual cases (Ackerknecht 1967, Foucault 1973) and in turn could be used to improve the accuracy of diagnosis. This allowed researchers to count similar cases of specific diseases and conditions.

But accurate studies of diseases in populations depend on numerators *and* denominators; that is, they require that cases of disease be compared with a completely measured population at risk. Diagnostic sophistication alone, which would only affect a numerator, was not sufficient. Methods of record-keeping to ascertain population denominators also were important. At about the same time that diagnostic methods were changing, so too were nation-states developing systems of record-keeping and vital statistics (Rosen 1955:39).

Finally, even as the body politic was being explored and constructed through census techniques, the interiors of individual bodies were being revealed via new technologies. The stethoscope appeared in 1819 in France, the compound microscope in the 1830s in England, the ophthalmoscope and the laryngoscope in the 1850s in Germany; and tissue staining at various sites in the 1870s. Each of these tools of observation and measurement created new classes of knowledge, and they allowed researchers to concentrate on more carefully defined categories of disease and agent. These new tools of measurement also narrowed the scientists' field of view: a wide-angled concern with the social environment tapered toward the end of the nineteenth century to focus on the biological. The analysis of pathogens largely replaced the analysis of poverty.

A.   Early Uses of Fieldwork in Epidemiology

Today, fieldwork is one of the hallmarks of training in anthropology. Anthropologists define themselves in part by where and how they do fieldwork. They do research among the homeless in New York City, in a town in rural Spain, on a plantation in Papua New Guinea, or in multiple sites, and they do it through long-term immersion and learning a local language, through a translator, or on short, intense visits. But fieldwork also has a longstanding tradition in epidemiology. In the mid-nineteenth century researchers did fieldwork to trace the origins and course of illness through populations. The best known of these investigations is probably that of John Snow (1855) on cholera. Snow has been called the prototypical field epidemiologist. His 1855 paper "On the Mode of Communication of Cholera" is a methodical, well-documented argument for a contagious and water-borne transmission of cholera. (The causal agent of cholera, the *vibrio cholerae*, would not be identified for another 30 years after this paper was published.)

Snow examined the pathology of cholera as a clue to the manner of its communication. For example, he noted that cholera infections commenced in the alimentary canal, and he reasoned that such a focus of first infection suggested that a substance had been ingested. He then presented examples of the spread of the disease in mines, row houses, and entire neighborhoods, and in this process he isolated important factors in the transmission of the disease. Snow mapped the topography of a cholera outbreak near Cambridge and Broad streets in London by means of a painstaking door-to-door survey, and he isolated the probable source of the epidemic to a particular well. His subsequent removal of the Broad

Street pump handle as a preventive measure has taken on great historical and symbolic significance.

Fieldwork like that performed by Snow was undertaken as part of the struggle between *miasmatists* (who believed that epidemics were caused by decaying matter circulating in the atmosphere) and *contagionists* (who believed that epidemics were caused by infectious organisms spread by contact or vapor, or via contaminated articles). With each group continuing to marshal empirical evidence in support of its theories, fieldwork became a common way to investigate the health effects of the environment in the latter half of the nineteenth century (Ackerknecht 1948, Terris 1985). The term "shoe-leather epidemiologist" is used still to distinguish those who collect data themselves out in the community from those who use existing databases.

It is an ironic historical twist that epidemiologists were committed to fieldwork before anthropologists invented long-term participant observation. Nineteenth-century anthropologists were more concerned with the history of institutions and ideas than with going to the field to collect data (Asad 1994:57). Anthropologists really did not begin to see fieldwork as an essential part of their discipline until the late nineteenth and early twentieth centuries, with expeditions to the Torres Straits and the Pacific Northwest.

Peter Panum, a Danish physician credited with describing the epidemiology of measles, did significant amounts of ethnographic fieldwork during his mid-nineteenth-century investigation of the causes of a measles epidemic on the isolated Faeroe Islands. Although Panum had no anthropological training, his 1847 report illustrates how valuable fieldwork can be for researchers who work in unfamiliar environments. The report opens with a strong plea:

When a physician is called to work in a place where climatic and dietary conditions are different from those to which he has been accustomed, his first problem is to study the hygienic factors which affect the state of health of the inhabitants. It is, in fact, these hygienic conditions which contribute towards the development and frequency of some diseases and the exclusion or rarity of others, and which more or less modify the symptoms of every disease. (1940 [1847]:3)

Panum wrote a quasi-ethnographic account of his five-month stay on the islands, describing the geography, climate, vegetation, physical conditions, and mode of life of the Faroese (including food preparation, housing construction and layout, clothing style, and occupation). He included these and other social conditions as part of a catalogue of potentially relevant causes of disease, although he had no explicit theory of multifactorial causation.

The German physician Rudolf Virchow was among the first to link fieldwork more closely to explicit theories about the role of society in the causation of disease. Virchow's biographer wrote that his report to the government about a typhoid epidemic in the famine-ridden province of Upper Silesia in 1848 is "an unusual and original document. Its fine clinical and pathological findings are embedded into an amazingly competent 'anthropological' (sociological) and epidemiological analysis" (Ackerknecht 1953:15). Virchow blamed the government for the epidemic and famine; he prescribed education, freedom, and prosperity as lasting solutions, in addition to the short-term palliatives of food aid or new drugs. Like Panum, Virchow was able to make concrete links between social conditions and disease outcomes based on his physical presence on the site, doing fieldwork and careful observation.

B.   Social Causes of Disease and Death

Virchow also offered ideas about how social revolution influences epidemic diseases. He labeled as "artificial" those epidemics that concentrated among the poor, determined by living and working conditions, and as "natural" those that were more evenly distributed among social classes (Ackerknecht 1953). Social justice, education, self-government, separation of church and state – these would decrease artificial epidemics like those he had seen in Upper Silesia.

Whereas Virchow made social reform a political essential, a few decades later the French sociologist Emile Durkheim helped to create strong theoretical arguments for focusing on the social causes of disease. Durkheim's book, *Suicide* (1951 [1897]), argues that suicide can be analyzed as a patterned social phenomenon. It is not only a private decision or individual act of will but a social practice following stable patterns of number and type. Durkheim's contribution was important both for its message and its timing. He upheld the legitimacy of examining social causes of disease just when germ theory was starting to dominate epidemiological research. Although Durkheim is not cited often as a major contributor to the history of epidemiology, his insights into the collective and social forces that affect individuals foreshadowed most of contemporary social epidemiology (Krieger 2001, Trostle 1986a).

The popularity of including a broad range of social factors in studies of population health was waning by the last quarter of the nineteenth century, in part because clinical researchers were searching for single causes for specific diseases and in part because social researchers were more interested in the evolution than the function of society. Research on diseases such as tuberculosis, syphilis, and pellagra continued to include social factors because the role of human contact was so obviously critical to understanding disease transmission. But attention to the etiological influence of the social environment would not resurface until the third and fourth decades of the twentieth century, when chronic diseases such as cancer, heart disease, and diabetes began to dominate the industrialized world's disease profile. Chronic diseases were not as easily explained by single-cause models. In addition, national governments faced increasing pressure to provide adequate health services, so they began to sponsor research on how to design, provide, and assess medical care and prevention programs. Chronic disease epidemiology and community medicine thus helped to revitalize research on the health effects of society and culture, although contagious disease epidemics, like the influenza pandemic of 1918–1919, also helped to rekindle research interest in the host and environment (Gordon 1953:61, Kolata 1999).

The renewed interest in the social environment in the 1920s and 1930s did not include the political overtones and sweeping environmental and political changes that had been advocated in the mid-nineteenth century. This partly was because the successes of bacteriology provided more specific measures of intervention than had been available earlier. It also was because clinical medicine was a focus of hope for developing effective new treatments. National health insurance and/or national health services were generating increasing interest in Great Britain, the European continent, the USSR, the United States, and South Africa. Reform predominated over revolution; researchers developed new treatments and new health programs, and argued for new legislation, rather than pushing for dramatic social structural changes.

II.   Epidemiology and Medical Anthropology in Collaboration

A.   Returning to Social Medicine: A South African Experiment

One such experiment in constructing a national health service began in South Africa in the late 1930s, culminating in the founding of the Pholela (also spelled Polela) Health Center in 1940 and the Institute of Family and Community Health (IFCH) in 1945. Pholela was a small rural clinic where an interdisciplinary team of clinicians, epidemiologists, and health workers first worked out the ideas of community health care used over the next five decades. Pholela is to international primary care what the city of Framingham, Massachusetts, is to the epidemiology of heart disease: a place where pioneering methods led to critical new knowledge.

The Pholela project merits extended attention here because it was the first health-care service specifically designed to assess the health status of a community using social science and epidemiologic methods. It drew on those assessments to develop and evaluate a comprehensive multi-disciplinary approach to improving community health. Many of the assumptions guiding research at Pholela were similar to those explored by nineteenth-century proponents of social medicine: poverty and social class are important determinants of health; social and cultural change affect the transmission of illness; and group as well as individual interventions promote health and prevent disease. The editors of the major book about the project acknowledged these similarities, titling their book *A Practice of Social Medicine* (Kark and Steuart 1962).

Reflecting on the Pholela project a decade after its inception, the first medical director, Sidney Kark, commented on the gains made after the first year of the experiment:

The whole process of the health centre's development was one which reflected an increasing understanding of the individual in terms of his family situation, of the family in its life situation within the local community and finally the way of life of the community itself in relation to the social structure of South Africa. By this detailed study the centre had moved from the plane of vague generalization about the importance of various social forces to an increasing understanding of those forces in relation to health and disease as manifested in individuals. (1951:677)

The significance of Pholela was that connections between social relationships and health were made an essential part of daily health center practice (*Ibid.*). The staff of the health center used epidemiology, especially a socially oriented epidemiology, to develop and evaluate the practice of community-oriented primary health care (COPC). They focused on social and cultural factors in the growth and development of children, the social causes of sexually transmitted diseases, nutrition and health, and evaluation of COPC's effect on health status. It is remarkable that South Africa, home to one of the world's most repressive political regimes in the latter part of the twentieth century, was earlier the site of the most creative experiment in combining insights of social science and epidemiology to describe and improve human health.

The biographies of Sidney Kark and of Emily Kark, his wife, help to explain the origins of the anthropological aspects of their research. As medical students they were influenced strongly by their association with the South African Institute of Race Relations (S. and E. Kark: personal communication), and in 1934 they began the "Society for the Study of Medical Conditions among the Bantu." In 1939 Sidney Kark was selected by the Ministry of Health to head a new health center in Pholela, a small rural African community in the province of Natal.

The Pholela Health Center was a pilot project designed to deliver effective and appropriate health services to rural South African communities. From its inception the Center was concerned with the social and cultural life of the surrounding community. The first activities of the Center included meeting with tribal chiefs and elders to discuss the program. The staff also consulted women's groups, local missionaries, school teachers, and parents of schoolchildren. The community health educators made multipurpose home visits to educate the community, learn about local health beliefs and practices, and identify those people most responsible for the dissemination of news and new ideas. Health center staff created an innovative gardening program, wherein people were given seeds, taught how to grow new vegetable varieties, and shown how to prepare a variety of nutritious dishes that conformed with local preferences; in addition they created a cooperative seed-buying project and community market. Early clinical work included examining schoolchildren, initiating a general medical clinic, and establishing a maternal and child health program. An epidemiological survey was conducted door-to-door to ascertain the health status of the community. The combination of survey work and action programs led the team to develop the concept of community health diagnosis, which includes monitoring a community's health as well as identifying targets for intervention (Kark and Kark 1981).

The Pholela Health Center was very successful: in 1944 the South African National Health Services Commission recommended that more than 40 new health centers throughout South Africa be constructed and administered according to the Pholela model. The IFCH was created under S. Kark's direction to train staff for the new health centers, conduct research, and practice family and community medicine. The Institute included seven health centers; the one at Pholela was its rural community health center, and six new centers were established by the Institute in and around the city of Durban to serve communities of various incomes and ethnicities. Each of these centers provided primary health care and served as a source of information for cross-cultural comparative research on topics such as child rearing, infant mortality, and menarche.

The Karks continued their training in epidemiology and social science: in 1947–1948 they studied epidemiology at John Ryle's new Institute of Social Medicine at Oxford University, and they worked with E. E. Evans-Pritchard, Meyer Fortes, and Max Gluckman, the primary forgers of British social anthropology at that time. The Karks analyzed much of their Pholela data in Gluckman's methodology seminar and in discussions with Fortes and Evans-Pritchard. In that setting they were able to refine their ideas about a socially oriented epidemiology (S. and E. Kark: personal communication).

Though it began optimistically, by the late 1940s the attempt to develop a South African National Health Service was under siege, and conservative politics eventually led to its failure. The infamous apartheid policy began to be assembled in 1948 with the election of a conservative government. Activists and dissenters interested in social equity and social medicine were harassed by the government over the next few decades, and many decided to emigrate.

B.   The Human Resources and Intellectual Legacy of the IFCH

When the South African government closed the IFCH in 1960, it signaled an end to its experiment in social medicine. Nevertheless the ensuing diaspora ensured that the IFCH staff, ideas, and methods would spread around the globe. A list of IFCH members who emigrated in the 1950s and early 1960s reads almost like a *Who's Who* of late-twentieth-century research and action in social medicine and social epidemiology (see Davey Smith and Susser 2002, Trostle 1986b).

The Karks emigrated to Israel in 1959, and they were joined there by other IFCH staff who had been invited to serve in the expanded program at Hebrew University. They began work in what soon evolved into the Department of Social Medicine (later the School of Public Health and Community Medicine) at the Hebrew University-Hadassah Medical School in Jerusalem. The group's ideas on how to incorporate epidemiology and social science into the delivery of health services to communities were presented in texts such as *Epidemiology and Community Medicine* (Kark 1974) and *The Practice of Community-Oriented Primary Health Care* (Kark 1981). Their ideas about how to make epidemiology a functional tool of health center practice were included in *Survey Methods in Community Medicine* (Abramson and Abramson 1999) and *Making Sense of Data* (Abramson and Abramson 2001).

Other South Africans associated with the IFCH went to Uganda and Kenya, where they founded health programs emphasizing preventive medicine much as was practiced at the IFCH. Still others came to the United States to apply their IFCH experiences to work in community health centers and major universities. For example, Mervyn Susser and Zena Stein, health center physicians deeply influenced by their work in the IFCH in the late 1950s (Oppenheimer and Rosner 2002, Susser 1993), came to the United States via Britain and became central figures in the development of epidemiology and public health in the United States (Davey Smith and Susser 2002). Susser was editor of the *American*

Journal of Public Health, co-authored an important text in medical sociology, and wrote many fundamental books and articles on epidemiologic theory (e.g., Susser 1973, 1987; Susser and Susser 1996). Stein was a leader in analyzing the relationship between maternal age and birth defects, as well as an important early proponent of developing methods women could use to prevent HIV infection (Stein 1985, 1990). The work of the IFCH also attracted foreign nationals, two of whom were important to the growth of social medicine and social epidemiology in the United States. Anthropologist Norman Scotch spent 18 months at the IFCH doing research on the causes of hypertension among the Zulu (e.g., Scotch 1960, 1963b), and soon afterward he wrote one of the first reviews of literature in the field of medical anthropology (Scotch 1963a). Scotch, who eventually came to direct the School of Public Health at Boston University, devoted a significant part of this review to epidemiology. He asserted that epidemiology at that point was essentially a method that looked at the combined influence of biology, environment, society, and culture on human health. He reviewed the application of epidemiology to diseases like *kuru* in New Guinea, psychopathology among the Eskimo, and hypertension among the Zulu, pointing out the broad attention paid to social change as a causal factor in all these cases.

H. Jack Geiger did a clerkship at the IFCH when he was a medical student at Case Western University and later published with Scotch on social factors influencing arthritis and hypertension (Scotch and Geiger 1962, 1963). In the United States Geiger became influential in the social medicine and community health center movements (e.g., Geiger 1971) and was a co-founder of major antinuclear and human rights groups (Physicians for Social Responsibility and, later, Physicians for Human Rights). Geiger clearly acknowledged his indebtedness to S. Kark and his colleagues (1984:17). COPC was promoted as a workable goal for medicine in the United States, and more than 600 federally funded community health centers existed in the United States at the peak of this movement in the 1970s (Geiger 1993, Mullan 1982). Two other U.S. experiments in providing health care duplicated many aspects of the IFCH: the Navajo-Many Farms Project in the late 1950s (see Adair and Deuschle 1970) and the Tufts-Delta Health Center from 1965 to the present (see Geiger 1971). Like the IFCH, each of these also was designed to deliver health care to urban and rural populations, and each also developed innovative methods that combined the social sciences with medicine and epidemiology. COPC also was successful in many other countries (Susser 1999, Tollman 1994).

The ideas and methods initiated at Pholela and the IFCH thus were disseminated throughout the world, helping to spawn similar projects in other areas. Phoelela and the IFCH showed that a combination of epidemiologic and social science methods could better understand the extent of community health problems, direct the focus of curative and preventive measures, and evaluate the effectiveness of these measures. Perhaps most important from an anthropological point of view, the IFCH experience taught its staff the importance of gaining cultural understanding (Kark and Kark 1962). This emphasis can be seen clearly in many of the projects and publications that resulted after the project halted and its staff scattered, in particular, in the work of John Cassel.

C.   From Practice to Process: Unpacking the Social and Cultural Environment

For our purposes one of the major ideas to emerge from staff trained at the IFCH was a conceptual framework for analyzing the social and cultural processes relevant to health. This framework was developed by an interdisciplinary team at the University of North Carolina, Chapel Hill, led by John Cassel, a former IFCH physician/epidemiologist, and the team also included an anthropologist (Donald Patrick) and a psychologist (David Jenkins).

Cassel was a South African physician who had joined the Pholela Health Center in 1948. The importance of the Pholela experience to Cassel's later work cannot be overestimated. His close contact with the health problems of the Pholela community, and the fact that his own attempts at curative and preventive care sometimes met competition from traditional medical beliefs and practices, helped him to develop an interest in the social and cultural components of health. This interest is stated most clearly in anthropological terms in a chapter titled "Cultural Factors in the Interpretation of Illness: A Case Study" (Cassell 1962). This case study is presented "as an illustration of the insight provided by knowledge of the cultural patterning and social situation into behavior which would otherwise appear as a series of inexplicable unrelated acts" (1962:238). It describes how two related kin groups in Pholela managed cases of pulmonary tuberculosis, cervical cancer, and persistent headaches, and it shows how knowledge of a series of related witchcraft accusations helped explain the management strategies chosen by kin groups and a missionary who became involved in the case.

Cassel also described the importance of cultural understanding in the Pholela project in his lead chapter in Benjamin Paul's classic 1955 text, *Health, Culture, and Community*. There he analyzed the different levels of Zulu resistance to the Pholela staff's curative and preventive efforts. Attempts by the staff to change attitudes toward food; to increase production and consumption of vegetables, eggs, and milk; to treat pulmonary tuberculosis; or to combat soil erosion – each was met by a higher level of resistance. The male labor out-migration created by South African labor regulations brought syphilis and tuberculosis into the community and challenged long-term treatment regimes for working-age males. Local unemployment and population pressure, combined with traditional food preferences and land use patterns better adapted to another time and place, helped make soil erosion a serious problem and malnutrition a common diagnosis (Cassel 1955:35). Understanding which cultural patterns were easiest to modify allowed the workers at Pholela to target their efforts toward reasonable goals; knowing who held power in the community allowed them to focus their actions on potential change-agents. Measurable health improvements were seen throughout the course of the project, especially in infant mortality, incidence of infectious diseases, and prevalence of malnutrition.

Cassel left South Africa in 1954 to join the School of Public Health at the University of North Carolina (UNC) at Chapel Hill. There he developed a strong joint faculty in the social sciences and epidemiology. Researchers in North Carolina confronted a largely agricultural state in the process of developing a postwar industrial base. The impact of society and culture on health was not as dramatic or life-threatening there as it had been in Pholela. Nonetheless, the studies undertaken by Cassel and colleagues in North Carolina eventually showed the equally significant health effects of such diffuse social processes as social and cultural change and adaptation. Cassel's conceptualization (1976) of the effects of the social environment on host resistance is his classic work; one measure of its importance is that it has been cited more than 800 times since publication.

The interdisciplinary team Cassel led at UNC-Chapel Hill published one of the first papers in social epidemiology to separate explicitly the social system from the cultural system. Acknowledging the work of the anthropologist Clifford Geertz, the authors defined culture as "the fabric of meaning in terms of which people interpret their experience and guide their action," while they defined social structure (which they equated with society) as "the way that group life is ordered, the persistent and regular social relationships of people" (Cassel et al. 1960:945). These distinctions were used to differentiate between the appropriateness of cultural norms and three different forms of social organization within which norms applied: occupation, family, and social class. Specific hypotheses could be tested within each of these three arenas. This paper showed the growing theoretical sophistication of researchers in social epidemiology. With the increasing general acceptance of the etiological importance of the social and cultural environment, it became necessary to develop theoretical models that could account for the obvious complexity of this environment.

In 1960, Cassel's team proposed an epidemiological study of the changes in health status that might accompany changes from a rural agricultural to an industrial way of life. Designed to take place in a manufacturing plant in a small Appalachian town, the study would compare three groups of people: agricultural workers, first-generation factory employees, and second- and third-generation factory employees. The authors hypothesized that the first-generation workers, those experiencing the greatest cultural change, would have poorer health status than the other groups. They also hypothesized that less family solidarity and greater incongruity between cultural background and current social situation would be most closely associated with poor health and adjustment. The research confirmed many of their hypotheses (Cassel and Tyroler 1961). Using measures of general morbidity and of absenteeism due to illness, the results showed that the health status of the first factory workers to move into the industrial area was lower than the health status of factory workers whose relatives already had been employed in the factory.

Under Cassel's influence, two other research topics linked epidemiologists and anthropologists at UNC-Chapel Hill: the epidemiologic study of diseases not recognized by biomedicine and the protective effects of social support on health. The medical anthropologist Arthur Rubel used his training in epidemiology at UNC-Chapel Hill to develop studies of the Mexican folk illness *susto* (Rubel 1964). This was one of the first times that the methods of epidemiology were applied to disease entities defined according to non-Western categories in an effort to understand their distribution and cause, even if they did not fit biomedical assumptions.

The second theme was a series of studies that established the protective health effects of social support, such as marital ties, friendships, and membership in community organizations. This work from the early 1970s helped to demonstrate the importance of host susceptibility and resistance – that is, factors that either increase or decrease the likelihood that an individual will become ill. Social support subsequently became a popular focus for studies in social epidemiology (Berkman and Kawachi 2000, Berkman and Syme 1979), but the anthropological origin of epidemiological interest in social support has largely been forgotten.

The UNC-Chapel Hill research has had a profound impact on social epidemiology. If the South African contribution is typified broadly as understanding how to provide and measure the benefits of health care to communities, the UNC-Chapel Hill work might be typified as developing epidemiological strategies to measure the health effects of social and cultural change. The new social medicine practiced in South Africa had its roots firmly (and knowingly) planted in a nineteenth-century sociological epidemiology; the UNC-Chapel Hill research on the effects of social and cultural change had an unacknowledged affinity with this same nineteenth-century work. For example, Rudolf Virchow wrote that epidemic diseases were markers of cultural change. While considering the contemporary epidemics of the industrial world – cancer, heart disease, stroke, other chronic diseases, accidents – Virchow's words maintain their significance: "The history of artificial epidemics is therefore the history of disturbances which the culture of mankind has experienced. Its changes show us with powerful strokes the turning points at which culture moves off in new directions" (Virchow, Report on the Typhus Epidemic in Upper Silesia, quoted in Rosen 1947:681).

D.   Redefining the Social Environment through Medical Ecology

I have paid specific attention to the research developed by Cassel and colleagues because of its relevance to contemporary social epidemiology and because of its links to the IFCH and South Africa. But by highlighting the research produced by specific people, I risk ignoring the broader intellectual surroundings that nourish such work. One critical part of this context consists of the ongoing attempts made in the twentieth century to define and understand the etiologic influence of the social environment.

The collaborative work between anthropologists and epidemiologists that began in the late 1950s came at a time of redefinition in epidemiology: articles at the time stated the field of epidemiology was "returning in large measure to the physicochemical and sociological orientation of the first half of the 19th century, but on a much sounder scientific basis than was possible at that time" (Terris 1962:1375). A number of epidemiology textbooks in the late 1950s defined epidemiology as applying to any and all diseases, infectious or chronic, and also stated the importance of the social environment as a factor in disease. Early literature reviews in the developing field of medical anthropology also started to discuss epidemiology at about this time (see Caudill 1953, Polgar 1962, and Scotch 1963a). Explicitly and consciously, the two fields were converging.

In 1958 the first paper was published stating explicitly that the disciplines of anthropology and epidemiology had noteworthy parallels (Fleck and Ianni 1958). Perhaps because it appeared in a journal of applied anthropology, the paper provoked little comment by epidemiologists (Fleck: personal communication; Ianni: personal communication). It emphasized the social aspects of the research by Panum, Snow, and other nineteenth-century epidemiologists and also discussed the difficulties of modern-day collaboration between anthropologists and epidemiologists. One primary difficulty was that anthropologists working in applied sociomedical research were commonly included only as consultants: they had little control over the nature of the questions being asked and learned little about epidemiology. Another problem was that epidemiologists historically had been too concerned with disease agents: these authors had high hopes for what they called an emerging "neoecological approach" in epidemiology, which would place greater emphasis on multiple causality and the importance of the environment. They also emphasized the importance of disease classification to epidemiology by remarking that "[t]he epidemiologist must be and is a social anthropologist with his particular interest being nosology" (1958:39).

Fleck and Ianni were correct in their estimates of the power of the emerging ecological approach in epidemiology, although their hopes for significant increases in anthropological engagement in this work would not be realized for two decades. Medical ecology was defined in the 1950s as an analytical perspective that focused on "the study of the populations of man with special reference to environment and to populations of all other organisms as they affect his health and his numbers" (Audy 1958:102). This interest had grown rapidly during World War II, when geographers mapped disease distributions and ecological habitats as part of the battles fought against tropical diseases in South East Asia. A well-known medical geographer once proposed that the term "medical geography" be replaced with the words "human ecology of health and disease" (May 1978 [1952]:212). But medical geography emphasizes the spatial aspects of disease distribution, whereas medical ecology stresses the organizational aspects of disease distribution. In contrast to a medical geographer's questions about place and time, a medical ecologist might investigate the manifestations of a disease at different ecological levels – cellular, individual, community, or population – and would consider the interactions among these levels.

One important result of the exchanges among medical ecology, medical geography, and epidemiology in the 1950s was that researchers were given further theoretical justifications for including the social environment in the study of the distribution and determinants of diseases. One researcher wrote that "the notable addition to the content of epidemiology under the influence of ecology is in relation to the social environment" (Gordon 1958:351). A 1960 text titled *Human Ecology and Health* expressed similar ideas:

Public health has always been concerned with man and his environment and, in this sense, oriented toward human ecology – though in a somewhat limited fashion at first. Today, however, the significance and the meaning of the term *environment* have acquired new proportions. Environment in this sense includes, of course, not only the material and spatial aspects of man's world but the nonmaterial web of human social relations called culture which profoundly influences man's state. (Rogers 1960:vii, emphasis in the original)

This emerging interest in ecology and health had two outcomes relevant to our theme. First, anthropologists began to be used to gain entrée into the field. In 1965, for example, members from the disciplines of epidemiology, social anthropology, entomology, sanitary engineering, public health nursing, and laboratory science embarked on an ambitious international comparative research project at the Geographical Epidemiology Unit at The Johns Hopkins University, designed to study the ecology of disease in five developing countries. The project team eventually published studies from Peru, Chad, and Afghanistan (Buck et al. 1968, 1970, 1972). The role of the social anthropologist in these studies was to collect contextual socioeconomic and cultural data and to facilitate the acceptance of the project within each study area. A cross-culturally applicable interview schedule was designed and translated into the respective national languages. Key informants were interviewed to obtain information about the different villages and cultures. But despite mention of the type and schedule of agricultural work, recency of settlement, frequency of out-migration and in-migration, and rapidity of social change, few systematic attempts are made in these three works to link the social and cultural environment with the descriptive epidemiology of tropical diseases. The social and cultural information serves as context, but the research was undertaken more to describe this context than to analyze its relationship to human health and disease.

E.   The Social Environment and Mental Health

Although psychological studies are not a primary focus of this chapter, it is important to mention that the mental health effects of social and cultural disorganization were being studied in the 1950s and 1960s alongside studies of the physical health effects of culture change. Perhaps the most important group engaged in the study of social disorganization and mental health at that time was formed by psychiatrists, anthropologists, and epidemiologists associated primarily with Cornell University. The group included a large number of senior anthropologists, including Marc-Adelard Tremblay, Charles Hughes, Norman Chance, Jane Hughes, and Robert Rapoport. The project directors (Alexander and Dorothea Leighton) were psychiatrists who held joint appointments in the Department of Anthropology. The first stages of the project involved more than

12 years of community fieldwork in an area of Nova Scotia they called Stirling County. They determined the prevalence of psychiatric dysfunction by having clinicians interview residents, and they compared this prevalence across the communities when arrayed along a spectrum of social disintegration. In all, 33 people participated in anthropological work over the first 10 years of the project (Hughes et al. 1960:531), and the project continues to this day (see Murphy 1994b, Murphy et al. 2000).

The authors described anthropological data collection as part of "a total approach to the County and its communities" (Hughes et al. 1960:7). Anthropological data would help readers understand epidemiological findings, as they put it, "so that as rich a background as possible is provided for understanding the context of the varying tendencies with regard to both prevalence and type of symptom pattern" (*Ibid.*:8). In a tradition that we have seen extending back to Peter Panum almost 100 years before, the authors were involved as participant observers:

[M]embers of our team have variously lived as neighbors, have grown gardens, cut timber from their own woodlots, fished on the bays, hauled lobsters, held offices in societies, taught nursery school, participated in the weddings, christenings, and funerals of friends and in turn had these friends share with us our own joys in new marriage and the birth of babies, and our sadnesses and fear when confronting sickness and death. (*Ibid.*:7)

Given our reference to Rudolf Virchow as a key nineteenth-century figure in the history of anthropology and epidemiology, it is important to note that one volume of the Stirling County report (*The Character of Danger: Psychiatric Symptoms in Selected Communities*, 1963) is dedicated to Virchow's memory, and its title is extracted from his writing on how to differentiate pathological from normal physiological processes. Virchow wrote that pathological processes are hard to distinguish from ordinary life processes, even consisting, at times, of ordinary processes happening at the wrong time or place. The Leightons and their colleagues thought that psychiatric disturbances were similarly difficult to define through sites of brain lesions or psychodynamic theories about how the mind functioned, so they used Virchow's approach to malfunction to justify assessing psychiatric status based on the type, frequency, and duration of impairment posed by psychiatric symptoms (Leighton and Murphy 1997).

This project, and similar population-based studies of mental functioning, created an early precedent for the contemporary interest of epidemiologists in human communities and their effects on health. As noted earlier, they realized the importance of establishing close and enduring relationships with communities under study, much as any anthropological participant observer would. They also clearly described the need for collaborative work between anthropologists and epidemiologists.

The Leightons' studies of mental illness and the UNC-Chapel Hill studies of physical illness started in the 1950s, when anthropologists were becoming interested in the concepts of acculturation (Beals 1953) and culture change (Lange 1965). However, while theories about the nature and effects of social and cultural change became increasingly useful in social epidemiology (Cassel 1964) and psychiatric epidemiology (Leighton et al. 1963), the applied epidemiological studies that explored the health consequences of such change had little impact on further theorizing in anthropology until the 1990s (see Chapter 3).

III.   Continuity and Change in Twenty-First-Century Projects Integrating Anthropology and Epidemiology

Before thinking about the new issues facing anthropologists and epidemiologists at the beginning of the twenty-first century, it is important to recall the contemporary themes that already have received decades of attention. For example, the interdisciplinary exchanges between these fields four and five decades ago were based partly on the movement of epidemiologists from home to foreign terrain. Anthropology became more relevant and necessary when epidemiologists started working more often in cultural contexts they did not understand. This theme is still relevant today, although the uncharted terrain now includes a mixture of foreign territories and domestic communities. As epidemiologists have become increasingly involved in the design and implementation of intervention trials attempting to change human behaviors such as unsafe sex, smoking, and high alcohol consumption, their need and desire to understand communities and human behaviors has grown correspondingly (Smedley and Syme 2000).

The growth of an integrated approach joining anthropology and epidemiology also rests on disciplinary responses to social and cultural change. Increased migration and urbanization make it important to define and measure the health effects of these social and cultural processes; a mixture of epidemiological and other social science theory and method is required for this purpose. We human beings are modifying our ecological context through the rapid transport systems we invent, the forests we cut down, and the new medicines and poisons we produce. Familiar diseases such as hypertension and diabetes are spreading more generally across the planet, helped along by changing dietary preferences and levels of physical activity. War, violence, political repression, and inadequate services shift people into new areas, bringing new customs, new diseases, and new epidemiologic patterns. Good fieldwork continues to be important to understanding this changing context because it puts researchers in direct contact with what they otherwise have to imagine (Agar 1996).

Studies of how the changing social and cultural environment affects human health will continue to be of critical importance for the foreseeable future. No single discipline can develop the complex models needed to account for the interplay between the individual and the environment and the rise of diseases such as AIDS, SARS, E. coli O157-H7, and antibiotic-resistant tuberculosis. As we will see in Chapter 6, interdisciplinary collaboration to treat and prevent these diseases is just as critical as the collaborative work undertaken to understand their burden and their causes.

Some of the forces that will continue to facilitate exchanges between anthropologists and epidemiologists in the twenty-first century are related to the growth of disciplinary research tools and knowledge not all that dissimilar from that of a century ago. For example, innovative administrative procedures in the nineteenth century helped create health insurance schemes, national health care, and systems of vital statistics. Administrative processes today help enroll or trace study participants or maintain consistent procedures across multiple study sites; these make it easier to use complex research designs and to increase the volume of research containing both biological and sociocultural variables. These procedures also facilitate looking at patient enrollment or nonparticipation in research studies as sociocultural processes relevant to epidemiologic research.

New technologies that facilitate the processing of large amounts of data will obviously continue to push interdisciplinary or integrated research studies. Statistical procedures such as path analysis and nonlinear regression make analyses of multivariate relationships more feasible. This allows researchers to examine multicausal models of disease causation that include social as well as biological factors. Ever-faster computers, cheaper massive data storage, and more complex computer-based statistical packages support the new analytic techniques critical to today's social and cultural epidemiologic research. Combining geographic information systems and statistical procedures for modeling and graphing social networks makes new studies of human interaction and disease transmission possible.

Technologies make information easier to process, but they also help make things visible. As stated earlier in this chapter, techniques of imaging such as stethoscopes, microscopes, and tissue staining helped to create new disease categories and scientific disciplines in the nineteenth century.

Twenty-first-century technologies for seeing inside human bodies, testing for genetic anomalies, and decoding the human genome are creating similar opportunities for joint anthropological and epidemiological research. These technologies help change definitions of disease and disorder even as they also modify how humans are grouped into "healthy," "diseased," and "at risk" categories.

Increased recognition of mutual interests between anthropologists and epidemiologists will continue to promote more frequent collaboration and more closely integrated studies and programs. Both disciplines actively debate critical issues such as the sources of their theories, validity of their methods, and utility of their findings. Medical anthropology has come to use a broad range of qualitative and quantitative research techniques to describe illness in biological and cultural contexts (Dunn and Janes 1986). Cultural anthropologists have assessed the use of statistics in anthropology and have written about the differences between ethnographic and statistical representation (Asad 1994). In similar fashion, epidemiology has subfields open to collaboration with anthropologists, and epidemiologists have expressed interest in qualitative methods and interpretive modes of inquiry (e.g., Almeida Filho 1992, Béhague et al. 2002, Black 1994, Breilh 1994, Donovan et al. 2002).

Some new big questions prompt discipline-based critiques within and across anthropology and epidemiology. In Chapter 1, I presented a description of cultural epidemiology as a field of study concerned with how diseases are defined and measured as well as patterned. The type of intense reflexivity seen in anthropology also has been articulated by some epidemiologists in the past decade. They have started to ask explicit questions about whether their paradigms of disease causation might best be labeled as "causal webs" (Krieger 1994), "black boxes" of unknown complexity, or "Chinese boxes" of nested levels of organization (Schwartz et al. 1999, Susser and Susser 1996).

Anthropologists are asking questions about the epidemiological vocabulary and method that mark some departures from the past. For example, only in the past few decades have they asked what the meaning of "race" is when used as an explanatory variable in studies of human health and through what causal pathways it might influence human health. They are giving similar critical attention to words such as "stress," "lifestyle," "risk," "socioeconomic status," and "community." They are asking how best to measure the mental health problems of diverse groups in the United States (Guarnaccia and Rogler 1999) and internationally (Weiss 2001), and how feminist perspectives can inform epidemiology (Inhorn and Whittle 2001). The following chapter takes a more detailed look at these kinds of questions.

Understanding how human bodies react to the presence, status, and power of others is another theme now receiving integrated attention. Studies of the influence of social support on human health have been joined by studies of the effects of social networks on human physiology and health. One critical question is how the environment and disease burden of the surrounding population influence individual disease risk. Strong evidence that poverty is a cause of sickness and mortality is being buttressed by evidence that the widening gap between rich and poor is itself a major cause of poor health and death (Farmer 2003, Kawachi et al. 1999, Nguyen and Peschard 2003). This is of particular interest to anthropologists because both pathogens and ideas about pathogens are transmitted through populations. The tools and theories to understand these phenomena must be able to move between the intracellular and the interpersonal, tracing causal relationships among pathogens, behavior, power, and disease.

FOR FURTHER READING

Ackerknecht E. H. 1953. *Rudolf Virchow: Doctor, Statesman, Anthropologist.* Madison: University of Wisconsin Press.

Cohen M. N. 1989. *Health and the Rise of Civilization.* New Haven, CT: Yale University Press.

Hahn R. A. 1995. Anthropology and Epidemiology: One Logic or Two? In *Sickness and Healing: An Anthropological Perspective.* Pp. 99–128. New Haven, CT: Yale University Press.

Krieger N. 2001. Theories for social epidemiology in the 21st century: an ecosocial perspective. *International Journal of Epidemiology* 30:668–677.

Kunitz S. J. 1994. *Disease and Social Diversity: The European Impact on the Health of Non-Europeans.* Oxford: Oxford University Press.

Lindenbaum S. 2001. Kuru, Prions, and human affairs: thinking about epidemics. *Annual Review of Anthropology* 30:363–385.

Porter R. 1997. *The Greatest Benefit to Mankind: A Medical History of Humanity.* New York: W. W. Norton and Company.

Rosen G. 1958. *A History of Public Health.* New York: MD Publications.

Trostle J. A. 1986a. Anthropology and Epidemiology in the Twentieth Century: A Selective History of Collaborative Projects and Theoretical Affinities, 1920 to 1970. In *Anthropology and Epidemiology: Interdisciplinary Approaches to the Study of Health and Disease.* C. R. Janes, R. Stall, and S. Gifford, eds. Pp. 59–94. Dordrecht: Reidel.

———. 1986b. Early Work in Anthropology and Epidemiology: From Social Medicine to the Germ Theory, 1840 to 1920. In *Anthropology and Epidemiology: Interdisciplinary Approaches to the Study of Health and Disease.* C. R. Janes, R. Stall, and S. Gifford, eds. Pp. 25–57. Dordrecht: Reidel.

Trostle J. and J. Sommerfeld. 1996. Medical anthropology and epidemiology. *Annual Review of Anthropology* 25:253–274.

3 Disease Patterns and Assumptions: Unpacking Variables

Dr. Donald M. Berwick, a Boston pediatrician, said recently, "Tell me someone's race. Tell me their income. And tell me whether they smoke. The answers to those three questions will tell me more about their longevity and health status than any other questions I could possibly ask."

(Kilborn 1998:A16)

Dime cómo mueres y te diré quién eres.
(Tell me how you die and I will tell you who you are.)
(Paz 1993:59)

A pediatrician predicts health status and lifespan from aspects of North American social status and identity; a writer divines identity from manner of death. These opposite positions are actually based on the same premise: that selfhood and mortality are intertwined. Both claims rest on the assumption that there are systematic connections between how people live and how they die.

Of course, *any* pattern of relationships between causes and outcomes is based on an underlying set of assumptions, because assumptions drive the choice of measures that allow the pattern to become visible. The choice of what variables to measure both directs and confines attention. As one researcher put it, "We will consistently fail to observe what we do not seek to find" (Burrage 1987). This chapter explores how different health-related disciplines define and employ a few key concepts: person, place, and time.

I. The Origins and Meanings of Disease-Pattern Categories

It is an epidemiological axiom that data can be reported according to categories labeled *person, place,* and *time.* A popular text from the 1980s, Lilienfeld and Lilienfeld's *Foundations of Epidemiology,* begins this way: "Epidemiology is concerned with the patterns of disease occurrence in human populations and the factors that influence these patterns. The epidemiologist is primarily interested in the occurrence of disease by time, place, and persons" (1980:3).

What characteristics do scientists identify as falling within these categories, and what do they leave out? Some of the common variables that epidemiologists think of as belonging to the category *person* include age, sex, marital status, race, socioeconomic status, religion, and occupation. But each of these variables potentially represents multiple underlying processes. A variable such as age, for example, represents a biological process of growth and development as well as a social process of changing recognition of status and responsibility. A variable such as religion represents a set of conditions (presence of faith itself, behaviors dictated by church doctrine, access to social support, ability to attend services) as well as a routinely collected marker of social status. Without explicit theories linking underlying processes to measured causal variables, the categories are meaningless, and studies linking them to health outcomes are difficult to understand and compare.

Similar complexities exist within other categories of disease patterns. When researchers describe disease risk associated with *place* they include social or political boundaries such as neighborhood, state, region, and nation, but they also – intentionally or not – include geological or other physical environmental influences such as altitude, level of sunlight, fluoride or arsenic content in water, or particulate or carbon monoxide content in air. The social environment also can manifest itself spatially, as in population density and urban/rural lifestyle differences or in those place-based effects of social stratification such as quality of police, fire, schooling, or medical services. Other variables related to place could include aspects of the biological environment (presence of mosquitoes, spores, or toxic plants). Once again, some of these variables represent specific biological exposures (air quality, radiation, micronutrient levels in local food), whereas others cover more complex interrelated influences (mobility, job availability, and the quality of schools and medical services).

The category of *time* also covers a wide set of processes. Calendar time measured as days, years, or other periods plays its own role in disease distribution, measured through variables such as the time between moment of exposure and appearance of symptoms, or duration of infectivity, or age at onset, or life expectancy after onset. But the cultural practice of dividing time into weekdays versus weekends itself influences disease, since the meaning of these time periods structures activities like drinking, sexual activity, recreation, and work. Time can be a marker of biological influence: for example, in the seasonality of disease fluctuations due to underlying variations in number of mosquitoes (for malaria or yellow fever), ticks (for plague or Lyme disease), or infected raccoons (for rabies). Time also enters studies through so-called cohort effects, where people born during a certain period or of a certain age have similarly patterned illnesses. And time as history also influences health research, both through changes in diagnosis or terminology and through changing patterns of behavior (popularity of smoking, age at first sexual experience) or even the changing significance of specific life-cycle achievements. For example, getting married or obtaining a high school degree elevated the status of young adults more in the 1950s than it did in the 1990s.

The categories of person, place, and time sometimes overlap. Migration is perhaps the best example because it involves persons changing places over time. Studies of migrants have had particular force in the attempt to discover the causes of obesity, hypertension, and coronary heart disease. For example, comparing populations of Japanese men in Japan with Japanese men in Hawaii and California allowed researchers to hold genetic variability constant while looking at the effects of changing diet and other aspects of acculturation (Marmot and Syme 1976). In similar fashion, Janes (1990) was able to see the health effects of migration among Samoan migrants to California.

A.   Mixing Person, Place, and Time: Modernization, Cultural Consonance, and Blood Pressure

What processes actually change as social conditions change or as people move to places where they encounter new conditions? Some possibilities include accumulation of goods, wage labor instead of subsistence labor, more time in formal education, loss of so-called traditional values and communal knowledge, changing diets and levels of physical activity, and acquisition of new norms and values. Studies by John Cassel and others proposed that changes in social conditions (urbanization, economic development, migration) led to greater stress and higher blood pressure.

Anthropologists and epidemiologists have investigated the health effects of such processes in numerous sites around the world, paying particular attention to migrants because they can be compared with those who stay at home (a baseline population) and because migrants usually change their behaviors and values as part of their adaptation to new sites. These studies show that the average blood pressure in the population tends to increase with modernization. These differences persist even when age and obesity are taken into account; they also tend to be larger among males than among females.

In attempting to understand discrepancies in hypertension rates between groups in complex, industrialized societies, anthropologist William Dressler and colleagues use the concept of "intracultural diversity" to emphasize that not all people who share a culture attach the same meanings to events or conditions (Dressler et al. 1996). What looks like a golden opportunity to one person might look like unseemly self-promotion to another, and the attributes and trappings of success also vary from person to person. Dressler argues that the existence and perception of stratification can have measurable health consequences; much of his work uses hypertension as a proxy measure of overall health.

Dressler is following some of the connections between social stratification and health that have been explored by the social epidemiologist Richard Wilkinson (1996) and others (Davey-Smith et al. 1990, Kawachi et al. 1997, Marmot et al. 1991). For example, Wilkinson argues that relative poverty, the size of the gap between rich and poor, not absolute poverty, is what best predicts high mortality and reduced life expectancy in industrialized countries. Unlike Wilkinson, Dressler explores what he calls "lifestyle incongruity": the health-reducing effects of attempting to maintain an unaffordable lifestyle (Dressler 1999). The flip side of "lifestyle incongruity," called "cultural consonance in lifestyle," measures the extent to which individuals are able to live in accordance with locally defined material standards.

In a series of studies of rural-to-urban migrants in Brazil, Dressler and colleagues first established which components of a material lifestyle were locally defined as most important, then whether people were able to achieve those ideals (1996). They found that blood pressure declined systematically as "cultural consonance in lifestyle" increased. They have also showed that the negative effects of "lifestyle incongruity" can be mitigated by strong social networks. Blood pressure is consistently lower – across societies – among individuals who enjoy good social support, even though the types of avoidance and coping strategies people use to deal with social and psychological pressures vary from place to place (Dressler et al. 1997). They posit that the fit between lived experience and perceived community standards has direct and indirect beneficial effects on blood pressure.

Dressler's paradigm offers an alternative response to those eager to see anthropologists map cultural groupings for epidemiologic purposes. Even if the boundaries of cultural areas cannot be defined with any precision, it is still possible to include these types of "cultural consonance" measures to determine who in a group holds shared values. This information can then be used to define group membership along the lines of present status, belief, or practice rather than residence within a zone of presumed like-minded souls.

B.   Connecting Person, Place, and Time: Disease Clusters

Epidemiologists must sometimes investigate whether the appearance of disease among a group of people in a delimited space at a particular time represents levels of disease greater than expected. One famous contemporary disease cluster is the child leukemia cases found in one neighborhood in Woburn, Massachusetts, popularized in the 1995 book and subsequent film called *A Civil Action*. Another is the illnesses and deaths in 1976 among a group of American Legion war veterans meeting at a hotel in Philadelphia, which gave rise to the name Legionnaire's Disease. Clustering of disease in one place is often thought by the public to indicate an infectious or environmental cause (air or water pollution, radioactivity, or energy from high-tension power lines), but epidemiologists and biostatisticians recognize that some disease clustering can be expected to occur just by chance, with no underlying common cause (Schinazi 2000). Clusters are not always easy to identify. For example, the movement of people into and out of areas creates complex and confusing exposure dynamics: a group of residents at any one time may include a few recent arrivals with only brief exposure to local environmental risks, and it will exclude those with long exposure who have already moved.

Disease clusters offer another opportunity to see the interplay among person, place, and time. Yet the very concept of a "cluster" depends partly on a series of political and social conventions. The way that boundaries are drawn around administrative space can determine the denominator. For example, six cases of childhood leukemia counted within a residential block looks more like a cluster than six cases in a census tract or town. These conventions also affect which diseases are thought to be rare, based, for example, on individuals or governments deliberately misleading people about disease status. Social interactions may influence whether knowledge of common diseases is shared in the first place (illness reported within members of a church or students in a school versus illness unknown because it occurs among isolated or marginalized individuals). Finally, political and social conventions influence the period of time over which a cluster is studied, as well as the duration and intensity of data collection. For example, when the SARS (Sudden Acute Respiratory Syndrome) epidemic was identified in early 2003, Toronto officials reported cases accurately but lobbied hard against World Health Organization (WHO) travel warnings imposed on their city, while Chinese authorities suffered devastating consequences for a much longer period of time as a result of lapses in surveillance and their unwillingness to report cases candidly to international health agencies.

II.   Assumptions about Defining and Measuring Variables

I have described two different levels of categorization of variables in the last few paragraphs. Person, place, and time represent very large group-ings of variables, whereas concepts such as religion, altitude, or season are more specific. But another aspect of measurement is also signifi-cant, namely, the specific question or measure used to collect information about a given variable called the operationalization of that variable. Con-sider, for example, how to measure the impact of "religion" on health status. Let's imagine a hypothetical experiment to assess the effects of religiosity on health. We might want to compare the health of people who pray with those who do not or the health of people who are prayed for with those who are not. (For a wonderful example of a test of this theory, see an 1872 paper by the statistician Francis Galton titled "A sta-tistical inquiry into the efficacy of prayer.") The investigator in this case would want to measure the frequency and duration of prayer. But would the results necessarily be valid? Perhaps the association between health status and religiosity could be equally well assessed not by the quan-tity of prayer but by particular health-enhancing behaviors associated with religious practitioners. Seventh Day Adventists, for example, who do not eat meat, smoke, or drink alcohol might be healthier than their nonreligious counterparts regardless of their prayer habits. Should re-ligiosity be measured by prayer, behavior, church attendance, or some other characteristic? Each measure might yield different conclusions about the effect of religion on health (Levin 1996).

The term "auxiliary measurement theories" has been developed to la-bel links between theory-based concepts and the indicators used to mea-sure them (Blalock 1968). Auxiliary measurement theories accompany the "definitions, assumptions, and propositions" that are contained in general theories being tested in any research study (Blalock 1990:24). For example, measuring religiosity through prayer rather than church at-tendance involves an auxiliary measurement theory that links religiosity to performance of faith rather than physical presence and network develop-ment in a house of worship. Unlike measuring whether there is an associa-tion between religiosity and health, assessing whether church attendance is the best measure of religiosity cannot be tested in a study. These aux-iliary theories guide the selection of specific variables and measures that are said to represent the underlying theory. Because they justify and guide the selection of measures, auxiliary measurement theories are an essen-tial part of any quantitative study design, although they usually receive little scrutiny. As I will show in the remainder of this chapter, one mean-ingful way anthropologists and epidemiologists collaborate is through "unpacking" the auxiliary measurement theories and the unexamined social and cultural components of common epidemiologic variables. In the following examples, I will begin to illustrate this process by unpacking the categories of person, place, and time.

III.   Aspects of the Category *Person*

Many different population attributes are categorized under the cate-gory *person*. The most obvious of these are age and sex, both associated with a wide range of illnesses. Other components of human existence classified under the category person include aspects of social position (occupation, wealth, education), human behaviors that increase or re-duce health, and physical attributes relevant to health status (nutritional status, height and weight, blood pressure). More recently, social epidemi-ologists have developed population attributes that cannot be reduced to individual characteristics: these include extent of income inequality in an entire group or systematic differences between individual aspirations and the resources available to achieve them. The following sections explore a few of the variables categorized under the category person, highlight-ing areas and studies where anthropology and epidemiology make joint contributions.

A.   *Status, Sex, Age, and Accident Mortality*

During an epidemiology course for medical students at the University of California at San Francisco in the early 1980s, Professor Virginia Ernster presented the class with a set of mortality data from what she described merely as "an unusual event." In a task reminiscent of the quote from Octavio Paz at the beginning of this chapter, the assignment was to use the distribution of the attributes of those who survived and died to guess what the event was.

The tables in this chapter summarize those mortality data from a num-ber of perspectives. Tables 3.1 and 3.2 show that males died in larger proportion than females, those of low or "other" social status died in larger proportion than those of higher status, and adults died in larger

Table 3.1. *Mortality by economic status and sex*

Economic Status	Population Exposed to Risk			Number of Deaths			Deaths per 100 Exposed to Risk		
	Male	Female	Both	Male	Female	Both	Male	Female	Both
I (high)	180	145	325	118	4	122	65	3	37
II	179	106	285	154	13	167	87	12	59
III	510	196	706	422	106	528	83	54	73
Other	862	23	885	670	3	673	78	13	76
Total	1731	470	2201	1364	126	1490	80	27	67

Source: Dawson 1995.

Table 3.2. *Mortality by economic status and age*

Economic Status	Population Exposed to Risk			Number of Deaths			Deaths per 100 Exposed to Risk		
	Adult	Child	Both	Adult	Child	Both	Adult	Child	Both
I (high)	319	6	325	122	0	122	38	0	37
II	261	24	285	167	0	167	64	0	59
III	627	79	706	476	52	528	76	66	73
Other	885	0	885	673	0	673	76	–	76
Total	2092	109	2201	1438	52	1490	69	48	67

Source: Dawson 1995.

proportion than children. Social and cultural hierarchies apparently seemed to preserve high class over low, and females and children over males and adults. Tables 3.3 and 3.4 show us the joint effects of social and cultural hierarchies on survival.

Data from Table 3.1 and 3.2 are summarized so that the proportion surviving within each subgroup is represented. Data from Tables 3.1 and 3.2 are summarized in Tables 3.3 and 3.4 so that the differential survival effects of the three major variables (economic status, age, and gender) are separated out. Comparing Tables 3.3 and 3.4 shows that survival (1) decreases as economic status decreases, (2) is higher for children than adults, and (3) is higher for women than men.

The event was the sinking of the passenger ship *Titanic* on its first voyage in 1912, when an iceberg tore open a series of watertight compartments. The boat was considered unsinkable, not enough lifeboats

Table 3.3. *Survival percentages separated by characteristics*

Male			
	Economic Status	Adult	Child
	High	32.6% of 175	100% of 5
	Medium	8.3% of 168	100% of 11
	Low	16.2% of 462	27.1% of 48
	Other	22.3% of 862	–
Female			
	Economic Status	Adult	Child
	High	97.2% of 144	100% of 1
	Medium	86.0% of 93	100% of 13
	Low	46.1% of 165	45.2% of 31
	Other	87.0% of 23	–

Source: Simonoff 1997.

Table 3.4. *Observed survival percentages by variable*

Economic Status	Percent Survived	Age	Percent Survived
High	62.5% of 325	Child	52.3% of 109
Medium	41.4% of 285	Adult	31.3% of 2092
Low	25.2% of 706		
Other	24.0% of 885		
Gender	Percent survived		
Female	73.2% of 470		
Male	21.2% of 1731		

Source: Simonoff 1997.

were available, and most of those who did not escape in lifeboats died. But note that two different rules about the value of human life shaped this pattern of mortality. Rule one is a social rule about class and status: higher-status passengers were preserved at the expense of lower-status ones, and passengers were saved before crew. (The economic status "other" refers to the crew.) Rule two is a cultural rule about gender and age: within economic status groups, females and the young survived at higher rates than males. This differential treatment marks the event as a maritime one, subject to the cultural rule of lifeboat access expressed as "women and children first." Would we similarly find better survival of women and children in disasters such as famines, for example, or in accidents such as large landslides or earthquakes?

The *Titanic* accident provides a simplified and stark example of the many pathways through which social and cultural meanings get translated into mortality patterns. Insufficient lifeboats was the result of what epidemiologists might call a faulty "environment" or a devastating design flaw that placed those on board at higher risk of dying. Social class stratification was manifested in the spatial separation of steerage passengers from high-class passengers who resided above the deck, and stratification by age and gender – pompously disguised as chivalry – determined that scarce lifeboat seats would be offered first to women and children.

The sinking of the *Titanic* is one of the most widely known examples in epidemiology of the force culture has in influencing how and when we die. A focus on the social epidemiology of *Titanic* mortality helps show the relationship between class and mortality, whereas a focus on cultural epidemiology points out how rules about the value of women, children, and crew in maritime accidents interact with rules about class.

B.   *National Assumptions about Social Worth: Vital Statistics*

The *Titanic* example shows how environment and sociocultural rules for behavior can create deadly patterns. But patterns also are created by bureaucracies that devise categories to describe individuals who have died. Systems of "vital" statistics (so-called because they refer to aspects of *vitae*, or life) do some of this work. There have been global standards for collecting vital statistics since 1900. Vital statistics allow patterns in the deaths of citizens to become visible but also – it should be remembered – to be obscured. Nation-states create patterned deaths in populations through their labels – their categorizations – of the dead. For example, infant mortality can be described by race, social class, or geographic location. Each category creates different patterns. Political states *form* their citizens' preoccupations even as they precisely quantify and measure their citizens' demise. The categories of state surveillance create vital statistics. This facilitates a conclusion that what one newly sees in vital statistics is somehow self-evident and natural rather than something created out of categories.

States create the conditions for life and death (Lock 2001). They also create meanings for, and memories of, those who die. In a sense, states breathe life into death; in Katherine Verdery's words: "Dead bodies have enjoyed political life the world over and since far back in time" (1999:1). Predictably enough, states categorize and value people who are dead at least in part according to the social worth they had when they were alive. Indeed, the state engages in a kind of mass obituary-writing exercise by the way it categorizes its citizens at death. The death certificate functions as a record of state priorities; it reflects and perpetuates conceptions of social worth and status, as well as domination and oppression. By deciding which social variables to record on the death certificate, the state makes judgments about the value of life, the causes of death, and the moral worth of individuals. In the process, it also steers health analysts toward specific understandings about the politics of death.

The death certificate serves the nation as the primary source of detail about those who have died. Because the international community agrees that standardization is necessary and useful, there are global conventions that govern the conceptualization, measurement, and recording of death. The World Health Organization has a committee that publishes worldwide standards (the latest version is called the International Classification of Diseases, Version 10, or ICD-10) for the types of information that should be collected on death certificates (World Health Organization 1992). Options range from summarizing income or wealth to describing skills, occupation, or economic relations (class) to labeling education, physical appearance, religion, or area of residence. The United Nations document "Principles and Recommendations for a Vital Statistics System" recommends that the following items are of highest priority in civil registration: cause of death, date and place of occurrence, age, place of residence, and sex (United Nations 2001). In addition, it also recommends these items with somewhat lower priority, occupation, literacy/ level of formal education, marital status, number of children, status as employer or employee, and age of surviving spouse.

Notwithstanding the existence of international standards, mortality data are processed and used locally. So even though all nations collect fairly similar data on their death certificates, countries can categorize and analyze those data quite differently. If systems of vital statistics manifest and form local prejudices, one should be able to see differences across nations in the way they are collected and how they are used to describe mortality. It is important to note, then, that despite the international recommendations for standards in collecting vital statistics through death certificates (WHO ICD-10), all nations do not measure the social status of their citizens in the same way. Even when they do measure the same way, they do not all analyze or present their information in a consistent fashion.

For example, Table 3.5 summarizes the social variables included in death certificates from a range of countries. Although many categories appear in the death certificates of all four of these nations, only the United States includes race and Hispanic origin, only Mexico includes citizenship, and only Argentina – and, since 2001, the United Kingdom – includes an assessment of employment status in addition to occupation (differentiating housewives from the unemployed,

Table 3.5. *Social variables included in death certificates from four countries*

| Variable | Country and Year of Last Revision of Death Certificate | | | |
	U.S.A. 2003	U.K. 2001	Mexico 1988	Argentina 2001
Age	√	√	√	√
Sex	√	√	√	√
Birthplace	√	√		√
Usual occupation	√	√	√	√
Occupational category				√
Industry	√			√ (Type of production)
Employment status		√		√
Hispanic origin?	√			
Race	√			
Citizenship			√	
Schooling	√ (Highest grade)		√ (Years and level)	√ (Years)
Marital status	√	√	√	√
Source of health insurance			√	
Habitual residence	√	√	√	√

Sources: Weed 1995; Ministerio de Salud, Argentina, 2001; Donkin et al. 2002; NCHS 2003; Instituto Nacional de Estadística Geografía e Informática, Mexico, 2003.

for example). In the United States, education was added to the death certificate for the first time as recently as 1989, explicitly as a surrogate for socioeconomic status (Tolson et al. 1991). The 2003 suggested revisions to the U.S. death certificate include a race category with responses ranging from "White" to "Asian Indian" to "Vietnamese" (National Center for Health Statistics 2003).

Almost all national data on mortality are first produced on a death certificate by a coroner, funeral director, or physician. But every country has varying levels of accuracy in completing the demographic portions of the certificate. For example, an evaluation of death certificates in South Africa found information on education missing from almost 47% of certificates, occupation insufficiently defined in 70%, and industry missing from almost 84% (Government of South Africa 2001).

Even when death certificates are filled out thoroughly, however, idiosyncrasies in analysis can result in different interpretations of the effects of social life on mortality. One common use of death certificates today is to make claims about the relationship between social status and mortality.

Many different types of measures of status are used, depending on what is available in the death certificate and what other types of census or survey measures can be linked to death certificates. But think about the variable "education" for a moment: it can be measured as "number of years of school" or as "degree or certification obtained" (Krieger et al. 1997). Measuring education as number of years implies that there is a constant increase in levels, such that the one year difference between sixth and seventh grade is the same as the difference between eleventh and twelfth. In contrast, education as degree or certification preserves the difference between completing primary school or not and, even more important in the United States, completing secondary school or not (*Ibid.*). These aren't right and wrong ways to measure education, rather they are right for some purposes and wrong for others.

The measurement of occupation is another place where auxiliary measurement theories play a role in vital statistics. Great Britain can use death certificate information to analyze how relative social position might influence mortality, whereas the United States is limited to analyses based on type of work performed. This is because the United States collects employment data based on usual occupation and industry. These data are summarized for almost all statistical purposes into 23 census groups that specify type of work performed *rather than* any measure of social or economic status (unless one were to argue that, for example, members of the major group "farming, forestry, and fishing" are of lower status than workers in the "transportation and material moving" group. [see the description of the U.S. Standard Occupational Classification System at: http://stats.bls.gov/soc/soc_home.htm]) The British also collect data on occupation, but their five primary occupational categories are arrayed along a spectrum of status and skill, from professional at one end to unskilled at the other, creating five levels of class.

Race is the variable most used to indicate social position in the United States, whereas class status indicates position in England. The more detailed categories of occupation in Argentina's death certificate might lead one to suspect that its statistics would be full of conclusions about work and mortality. But appearances can be deceiving here, too. In fact, through June of 2001 the list of official publications of the Instituto Nacional de Estadística y Censos (statistics office) of Argentina since 1984 still contains no title mentioning *any* social category other than province of residence as a covariate of adult mortality.

Although occupation data seemingly could be used for this purpose in Argentina, the socioeconomic portion of the death certificate in Argentina for the past few decades has been filled out quite haphazardly, if at all.

The national statistics office began a campaign in 2001 to increase the accuracy and completeness of data on the death certificate. In its vital statistics publications, the Argentine government expresses social position *only* through province of residence. These provinces have been categorized into zones of high, medium, and low resources, and are used as geographic indicators of social ranking (Verdejo 1998).

In Mexico's death certificate the variable "health insurance" provides one useful clue to social position because government workers are in one system, commercial workers in another, and oil industry or armed forces members in others. But Mexico as a nation attends most closely to social position based on ethnicity, separating indigenous from other citizens based on language spoken. Because language is not included in the death certificate, estimates of the mortality of indigenous groups are calculated from other sources, such as special surveys, or from death certificate data collected from municipalities with high proportions of indigenous-language speakers (see Sepulveda 1993).

Thus, national systems of vital statistics respond differently to calls for international standardization of death certificates. Not all recommended variables are measured, and some idiosyncratic ones, such as race, are added. Not all deaths are recorded, and the poor are less likely to be counted in death just as they are counted less in life (see Scheper-Hughes 1992). Even when categories exist on forms they are not necessarily filled out. And even when they are filled out, they are not necessarily analyzed or published. What is published tends to reflect, and constrain, national debates about forms of intervention and prevention. It seems natural to talk about race and mortality in the United States, but this is partly because for many years it was the primary variable offered by our vital statistics system to measure social stratification. Social epidemiologists in the United States who wish to look at how class position influences mortality still cannot use death certificate data for this purpose because the occupational categories used cannot easily be transformed into measures of class position. Epidemiologists and decision makers in Argentina are even further distanced from identifying specific groups at high risk because these differences are presented only as geographical differences.

The most important point about all these varied measures of social position is that people of lowest status have higher infant and adult mortality. Whether one looks at mortality rates of people ranked by province, class, occupation, or language, lower status consistently predicts higher mortality across nations. The pattern of death is the same in each of these nation-states no matter what conventions of measurement have been selected. But some death certificate forms make this easier to spot than others; some countries do not have the procedures or enforcement required to make their data useful, and others let categories like race or indigenous language serve as a proxy for social class. These are some of the cultural influences on the statistics as well as the causes of mortality. The next section looks more closely at one particular status measure, namely race, as employed in United States health statistics.

C.   Race as a Cultural Category and as a Risk Factor for Ill Health

The United States is one of the few countries that collects and uses race data on death certificates. But just what is race, and what does it mean? Despite the fact that race is commonly invoked in public health and medical literature, definitions of race are rare, conflicting, and muddled. Race is such a central concept in American culture that it can be seen practically everywhere in clinical and epidemiologic reports published in the United States. There was even a clinical volume titled *Textbook of Black-Related Diseases* (Williams 1975). Public health researchers in the United States often classify their populations by race, ethnicity, or national origin. These categories were used in just over 50% of the 914 articles on human populations published in the *American Journal of Public Health* (AJPH) between 1980 and 1989 (Ahdieh and Hahn 1996). Among the many research articles in the AJPH using racial and ethnic categories, only a small percentage (8%) included clear definitions of these terms. Race is included in research articles even when it is irrelevant to the disease explored: this was the case for 82% of the AJPH research articles, and 40% of 313 published medical case reports reviewed elsewhere (Negre 1985).

The rest of the world is not so obsessed with race as a marker: a review of online articles from the U.S. National Library of Medicine (MedLine) from 1990 to 1996 demonstrated that 80% of studies of infant mortality from the United States mentioned race or ethnicity, whereas only 22% of studies from outside the United States mentioned these two categories (Anderson and Moscou 1998). U.S. health researchers appear to pay extensive attention to these characteristics yet neither define them well nor use them consistently.

Critics of the use of "race" as a biological variable argue that it cannot capture and explain human variability. Genetic variation is widespread and gradual; no sharp geographic differences clearly separate racial groups. Genetic studies show conclusively that the variation within groups labeled as "White" and "Black" is greater than variation between those groups (Lewontin 1972) – so these labels give a false sense of group coherence.

Yet "race" is always grouped into a finite number of categories. Some of these still carry vestiges of nineteenth-century social and biological thinking about racial superiority (categories of Caucasian vs. Negroid vs. Mongoloid). Other racial categories are based on an arbitrary labeling of skin color as white versus black versus yellow versus red. Others are based on a combination of language, skin color, and national origin (White, Black, Hispanic). Still others, such as the five racial categories adopted by the United States government in 1997, combine skin color and geographic origin (White, Hispanic, Black or African American, Native Hawaiian or other Pacific Islander, American Indian or Alaska Native). This was the first time the government separated the ethnic category of language (Hispanic) from the other racial categories, allowing it to be applied to all of them. But what sort of human variability is being measured if the categories include both skin color and geographic origin, are based on self-assessment, and change over time?

Besides, genetic variation exists in many characteristics other than skin tone, and there is no packet of physical characteristics that varies consistently with skin tone. Classifying people into races based on skin color is as arbitrary as choosing hair color, nose shape, or earlobe size – no single physical trait can encompass human diversity. The clinical consequences of racialist assumptions can be quite serious. For example, when the genetic disorder that causes sickle cell disease is thought to be confined to people of African ancestry, a "White" child entering the emergency room suffering from sickle cell-induced hemolytic crisis may not be diagnosed as readily as she would have been if she were "Black." Because the sickle cell trait was an evolutionary response to the presence of malaria it became distributed among populations exposed to malaria, including those in southern Europe, India, and the Middle East. The gene is distributed along geographic, not racial, lines, but racialist thinking can exacerbate the social toll exacted by sickle cell disease.

The U.S. federal government officially began to acknowledge the complexity of human mixing when it allowed people to select multiple racial categories on the national census forms in 2000. About 6.8 million people, or 2.4% of the United States population, reported during the census that they belonged to more than one race (U.S. Bureau of the Census 2001b). Those reporting more than one race tended to be younger than those reporting just one race, reflecting how these identity choices can change over generations. Among those younger than 18, 34% of respondents saying they had one race also reported Hispanic or Latino origin, whereas among those reporting two or more races, the proportion of Hispanic or Latino origin was 43%. If racial classifications change from one generation to another, the public health outcome is an inability to compare "racial" measures from early studies with those from later ones.

Race is such a central component of identity in the United States that researchers include it almost by default. Proponents of racial categorization argue that it is a proxy for genetic variation, however imperfect, and that it *is* empirically correlated with health problems ranging from cardiovascular disease to diabetes, cervical cancer, lead poisoning, and handgun deaths. The presumed connection between race and genetics is frequently taken to extremes, leading some researchers to attribute differences in IQ scores, sports performance, and health indicators to race rather than to the effect of race in a racist society.

Anthropologists argue that race is a social category, not a biological one (Armelagas and Goodman 1998, Goodman 1997, Tapper 1999). Racial discrimination against Blacks still limits opportunities, reduces inherited wealth, and creates health-reducing discrepancies between aspirations and status. Being "Black" in the United Status does not mean having different genes than being "White" because there is more genetic variation within each group than between them. But it does often imply having lower economic status, lower educational attainment, reduced access to health and housing services, exposure to environmental contamination, inadequate or nonexistent health insurance, and differential treatment by police and health personnel, to name just a few dimensions. Rather than marking genetic difference, then, the variable called "race" marks a broad range of concepts extending from stress and discrimination to physical environment and diet. "Race" is social rather than biological and carries many different meanings. (To emphasize the social content of "race," from here on I will refer to the concept and to individual racial categories using quotation marks.)

If "race" has such poor theoretical foundations and is impossible to define or measure well, why does it continue to be so widely used in public health and medical research? There is a legitimate argument for continuing to include "race" as a component of epidemiological research: even though the biological basis of "race" has been thoroughly discredited, the social uses of "race" continue to have biological effects. In a racially stratified society, "race" sorts people into social categories and sets them on different life trajectories. This in turn influences their earning potential, educational achievement, access to health services, occupation, and lifestyles, which result in definite and measurable biological outcomes. In order to identify and intervene in health disparities, it is therefore sometimes useful to collect information by "race," if only to see the effects of racism. The problem emerges when the category of "race" gets used uncritically to classify categories of people. Such pigeonholing reinforces and perpetuates the impression that health problems are linked only to biology rather than to histories of oppression and continuing racial discrimination. Pigeonholing can foster a tendency to blame the victim, by implying that health disparities are located in "race" instead of in racism. Rather than continuing to rely on "race" as a characteristic of individuals or groups, it would make more sense to investigate the social effects and biological consequences of racism. The next section explores and critiques the assumptions governing the broad use of "race" as a predictive variable in public health.

MEASURING IDENTITY AND ORIGIN

Federal agencies do a poor job of defining and measuring race, ethnicity, and national origin. According to medical anthropologist Robert Hahn (1992), the variable "race/ethnicity" misses all four key qualities required of variables if they are to be good choices for use in national statistics.

1. Categories must be consistently defined and ascertained. Hahn shows that respondents and observers classify "race" differently, even though the census says race is determined by self-identification. He and his colleagues analyzed data from the National Health and Nutrition Exam Survey to see how ethnic identity changed after 10 years:

- 42% of respondents specified a different primary ancestral identification at follow-up;
- 15% gave a primary identification at the first interview that did not match any of up to four ethnic backgrounds they gave at the follow-up interview; and
- 45% of proxies (comprised predominantly [89%] of spouses, roommates, children, and siblings, and 11% by nonrelatives) gave a different primary ancestry for subjects than the subjects themselves had given (Hahn et al. 1995:79).

2. Categories and designations are understood by the population being counted. Hahn and others (e.g., Hahn and Stroup 1994, Mays et al. 2003) have documented that racial and ethnic categories mix categories of geographic origin (Pacific Islander) with labels of skin color (Black/White) and ethnic categories based on shared characteristics of language and culture along with geographic origin (Hispanic, Native American, Asian). These categories periodically get changed by government agencies, and they have no necessary correspondence to populations' self-perception.

3. Enumeration, participation, and response rates are high and similar for all racial and ethnic populations. For vital statistics to provide valid estimates of subpopulations, those subpopulations must have equal chances to be counted. Yet Hahn cites data showing that births are under-registered for some groups, "race" is misclassified at death for some groups, and both miscounting and survey nonresponse rates differ among "racial" and ethnic groups (Hahn 1992).

4. *Responses of individuals are consistent in different data sources and across time.* Hahn and colleagues investigated the racial classification of U.S. infants (age less than one year) who died between 1983 through 1985 and whose birth and death certificates could be linked. In this group, "race" noted at birth differed from "race" noted at death among 3.7% of the infants (Hahn et al. 1992:261). The size of this difference varied greatly by "race": it changed among 1.2% of infants classified "White" at birth, among 4.3% of those classified as "Black" at birth, but among 43.2% of those with a racial classification other than "White" or "Black" at birth. And these infants whose racial classification changed largely became "White": the number of infants classified "White" at death was 2.5% higher than at birth, whereas the number classified "Black" at death was 1.9% lower than at birth, and the number classified "Filipino" was 44.5% lower than at birth (Hahn et al. 1992:261). Because the number of misclassified infant deaths is higher in these "non-White" groups, the real rates of infant mortality for "non-Whites" are even higher than estimated.

In summary, public health researchers in the United States often stratify citizens by "race" and use this label even when it is undefined and irrelevant to the subject at hand. Being one among many components of identity, racial classifications change over time and are rarely well-bounded or well-defined. Used as an analytic category for public health purposes, "race" mixes personal with environmental characteristics, maintains stereotypes, and provides illusory risk information. Using "race" as a marker of disease patterns makes little sense because it reinforces the confusion between social and genetic causes of illness. In this case, poorly justified indicators provide support for ill-defined concepts.

Some public health practitioners have argued that "race" can be used as an indicator of social rather than genetic difference. They note that "race" is unquestionably associated with health differences, but that it is a marker of experience rather than genetic make-up (see Jones 2001, in a commentary that discusses how to use "race" in epidemiologic practice). Kaufman and Cooper (2001), for example, point out that aspects of diagnosis and treatment that may be related to "race" or ethnicity can and should be studied. This can be done by using actors or sample records to vary "race" and ethnicity systematically when presenting medical cases or records, while holding constant other aspects of identity and disease. Researchers can thereby uncover the specific health-related influence of *ideas* about "race" and behaviors toward different "races." These authors recommend continuing to use "race" or ethnicity cautiously as a part of monitoring disparities in health care and disease rates over time. They also recommend using it where "race" or ethnicity might influence social interactions between patients and health services. But they do not recommend using racial or ethnic variables in studies of disease causation.

D.   Determining Who and What Gets Counted

Another aspect of the category *person* consists of decisions about who should be included as a case. Case definitions are critical components of epidemiologic studies – they determine how many cases will be compared with a population total. Arriving at valid diagnoses in cross-cultural epidemiologic studies requires accurately and consistently defining cases, but this is a source of debate between some anthropologists and epidemiologists. The basic concerns from the anthropological side are with the legitimacy of applying Western disease categories to non-Western groups, the accuracy and validity of using large-scale surveys to assess health status, and whether the complexity of culture can be reduced to a set of predictive variables. One example of this controversy grew out of the 1950s and 1960s collaboration between psychiatric epidemiologists and anthropologists studying the relationship between culture and mental status in the Stirling County studies (see Chapter 2). As psychiatric epidemiologists grew increasingly interested in establishing clear and consistent case definitions across different cultures, a strong critique of epidemiologic categories developed in the 1990s, labeled "the new cross-cultural psychiatry."

Is it better (more valid and effective) to use varied local definitions of mental status or consistent but foreign definitions? Advocates of the new cross-cultural psychiatry propose that the concept of culture be used more as a description of context than as a type of causal agent in epidemiologic studies of mental status. The difference can be seen in the contrasting viewpoints between the psychiatric epidemiologist Jane Murphy and the anthropologist Byron Good. Murphy pleads for anthropologists to "prepare maps and draw boundaries so that cultural areas can be identified where certain beliefs are widely if not universally subscribed" (1994a:54). Good, by contrast, argues for "more explicit focus on local social and cultural environments" (1997:243). Murphy wants anthropologists to make it easier to categorize population denominators by drawing clear boundaries among cultural groups; Good conceives of culture not as geographically bounded but rather as starting from "heterogeneity, stratification of power and wealth, and contested claims" (1997:243). These changes in the concept of culture have prompted anthropologists to become more critical of epidemiologic perspectives that would employ culture as a risk factor like any other (DiGiacomo 1999).

Culture also is coming into vogue in biomedicine as doctors discover how culture affects clinical encounters, doctor-patient communication, and compliance, as well as the health profiles of populations. Greater attention to culture cannot but be positive in a multicultural society, where a long history of biomedical dominance has spawned a huge industry of alternative and complementary health practices. By asking about people's understandings of disease etiology, best treatment, correlates, and likely outcome, physicians can better appreciate how to treat patients and prevent disease. This is the logic behind the "cultural competency" movement, in which medical students and practicing professionals are trained to recognize and handle cultural difference. But culture is too easily oversimplified, and one pitfall of the cultural competency movement is that it tends to locate culture "out there," in patients (see the warnings in Denberg et al. 2003). Culture is not a list of traits, nor should anyone assume that ethnicity, language, or religion are accurate indicators of belief. Some of the more egregious cultural competency formulations ignore the fact that we are all immersed in culture and that biomedicine has culture, too.

Medical training in "cultural competence" is one example of the tension between defining culture as an assemblage of traits and defining it as a set of contested meanings. An online publication called "The Provider's Guide to Quality and Culture," from the Manager's Electronic Resource Center (available online at: http://erc.msh.org/), in 2002 described the health-related "strengths and protective factors" and "dimensions of vulnerability" for five different groups in the United States, labeled as "African Americans, Asian Americans, Hispanics/ Latinos, Native Americans, and Pacific Islanders." By 2004 it had added four more groups. This website is plastered with warnings "not to stereotype," but from an anthropological perspective it looks like a crude cultural cookbook that equates ethnic identity with specific health beliefs and behavior. Notice that some of these five groups are labeled by geographic origin and others by language. One could be left with the mistaken impression that the "Asian" origins of upper-class Pakistani Muslims, middle-class Thai Buddhists, and working-class Spanish-speaking Catholic Filipinos in the United States somehow give a common unifying identity relevant to their health status and behavior, and that the concept of culture maps neatly onto the ethnic and racial categories used only in the United States. The site's advisory notice that "the categories of regions and groups included here are somewhat arbitrary" (Management Sciences for Health 2004) does not address this concern.

If culture becomes oversimplified in this fashion, then those who follow these guidelines risk blinding themselves to variability, contingency, and struggle. If one starts to think that all Puerto Ricans, all Asian Americans, or all poor urban residents are the same by virtue of a common label, then one loses the ability to see how history, environment, and experience influence identity and behavior.

IV.   Aspects of *Place*

Variables categorized as *place* influence health in some relatively straightforward ways: the living organisms (parasites, viruses, bacteria) that cause most infectious diseases are often affected by place-based factors such as temperature and humidity. Parasites, for example, flourish in warmer humid places, and as such are a primary focus of so-called tropical medicine. Soil nutrients can be absorbed by humans through the consumption of crops: iodine-poor soils can cause goiter, and foods low in iron can cause anemia (Cohen 1989). Many international epidemiologic studies are now investigating the effects of site-specific Vitamin A deficiencies on blindness or zinc deficiencies on susceptibility to diarrheal diseases.

The influence of place can be seen easily in the distribution of *vector-borne* diseases such as malaria or yellow fever, both spread by mosquitoes. The maps in Figure 3.1 show changes over time in the spread of the *Aedes aegypti* mosquito, a major vector for dengue and yellow fever.

Place is complex in many of the same ways that person is. It can refer to aspects of the natural physical as well as the "built" (human) environment. It can include everything from water quality to crime levels, job availability, or exposure to chronic stress. Places influence patterns of health because they expose residents to systematically different qualities of the natural physical environment (e.g., ultraviolet levels in sunlight, or micronutrient levels in soil). But of course humans have modified many aspects of the natural physical environment: deep wells expose Bangladeshi villagers to high levels of arsenic in their water, and smokestacks push small particulate matter or sulfur dioxide into the air breathed by residents of Mexico City or Los Angeles. Neighborhoods have diverse sociocultural features, including varied politics, history, norms, threats, and networks. And they have varied reputations among residents, outsiders, and planners (Macintyre et al. 1993:220–221, Macintyre et al. 2002).

Anthropologists, sociologists, geographers, and epidemiologists are all trying to untangle the more subtle and complex ways that local area influences individual behavior and disease risk. As explained in more detail in the next section, intrahousehold patterns of behavior can influence who

1970   1997

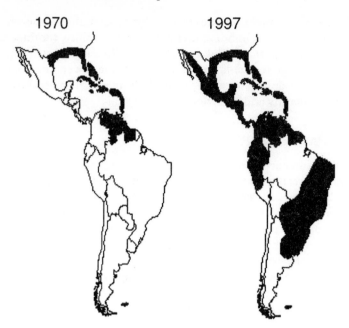

Figure 3.1. Distribution (shaded) of *Aedes aegypti* mosquitoes in the Americas in 1970, at the end of the mosquito eradication program, and in 1997. *Source*: CDC Division of Vector-Borne Infectious Diseases, available online at: http://www.cdc.gov/ncidod/dvbid/dengue/map-ae-aegypti-distribution.htm.

becomes sick in a family; but social exchange networks between families also can influence how pathogens travel, and movement of key individuals across networks can bring new pathogens to distant regions.

*A.   Through What Social and Cultural Pathways Does
       Place Influence Health?*

One way place influences health is through neighborhood of residence. Sociologists have documented that neighborhood characteristics influence how young children and adolescents develop. More specifically, they have shown in the United States that the presence or absence of affluent neighbors or classmates influences teenage birthrates, childhood IQ, and school-leaving (Brooks-Gunn et al. 1993); that neighborhood context influences young women's use of contraceptives and risk of nonmarital intercourse (Brewster 1994); and that it influences teenagers' probability of dropping out of school or having children (Crane 1991). Studies by epidemiologists have suggested that neighborhood social environment influences, among other outcomes, general mortality (Yen and Kaplan 1999a), risk for developing depressive symptoms and decline in perceived health status (Yen and Kaplan 1999b), and women's heart disease mortality (LeClere et al. 1998). Neighborhood may influence behavior and disease through prevailing social norms, exposure or protection from pathogens, and even attraction of people at increased risk of disease.

Because humans live in close proximity, each person is invariably influenced by many others. Like it or not, our ability to enjoy good health and survival is determined, to a considerable degree, by the beliefs, motives, and preferences of our neighbors (Granovetter 1978). For example, epidemiologists know that those who do not immunize their children are relatively safe from infection so long as a high proportion of the surrounding population continues to immunize. This "herd immunity" protects all members of the population regardless of their immunization status because overall protection is high enough to prevent isolated cases from widely spreading their infection.

Because we live in a society that favors autonomy and independence, we often act as though the risk of disease is independent for each individual. Yet in the preceding paragraphs I have argued that the risk for any one individual is often contingent on the behavior of others; for example, on the proportion of those who already engage in some health-reducing or health-enhancing activity or who have already been exposed to an infection or other insult (see Koopman and Longini Jr. 1994). People become increasingly likely to contract an infectious disease as the number of cases around them increases, or as they become increasingly likely to meet infected cases because of migration or by virtue of having similar practices. For example, the likelihood that an intravenous drug user will become infected with HIV increases as HIV rates increase among people with whom he or she shares needles, and the likelihood that a teenager will smoke increases as the proportion of her friends who smoke increases.

The social context of disease is particularly interesting to anthropologists because of the connections between social mixing (another aspect of place) and disease transmission. The average number of people one comes in contact with per day can influence exposure to infectious diseases. But so can the proportion of people one knows who in turn know and contact one another, as well as the number of intermediaries between one person and another within a network (Morris 1993, Wallinga et al. 1999). Population mobility can change all of these aspects of connectedness.

Two biological anthropologists, Lisa Sattenspiel and Ann Herring (1998), demonstrated these complex relationships when they studied historical data describing the 1918–1919 influenza epidemic in northern Canada in isolated Hudson's Bay Company posts linked by rivers. They used census data, company records of visits, and mortality records to help reconstruct both the visiting patterns among three trading posts and the spread of the epidemic. Mathematical models helped them to simulate what would have happened to the severity and timing of the epidemic if it had started at one or another of the three sites, if contact rates differed within communities and between communities, and if rates of travel differed among communities. They showed that the severity of the epidemic was determined primarily by contact rates within communities, whereas the timing of the epidemic was affected by contact rates within communities and by mobility patterns between communities.

Increasingly sophisticated theories and research methods are allowing joint aspects of place and person to be studied to explain patterns of disease transmission more fully. For example, an outbreak of tuberculosis in Houston, Texas, was studied using methods from molecular biology, epidemiology, ethnography, and network analysis (Klovdahl et al. 2001). Most epidemics of infectious diseases are investigated using so-called contact tracing, where an infected individual is asked to identify others who might have become infected. In this study, however, DNA techniques allowed the researchers to "fingerprint" the tuberculosis strains in the epidemic and thereby identify which people had been infected with a common strain. Interviewing patients uncovered only 12 person-to-person contacts among 37 infected people with an identical strain of tuberculosis. However, by combining network analysis with attention to places where these individuals might have been together, the researchers were able to show that at least 29 of these 37 people could be linked directly through other people or indirectly through places they frequented. Interdisciplinary teams such as these are combining their theories and methods to develop increasingly powerful, complex, subtle, and accurate models of place.

Another example of how categories of person, place, and time come together through ethnographic studies involves an investigation of how local context influences needle-injection practices and risk of contracting HIV. As part of a multi-site study to understand and reduce AIDS and hepatitis risk among intravenous drug users, an interdisciplinary team of epidemiologists, anthropologists, and microbiologists (Singer et al. 2000) used a broad series of qualitative methods to understand how neighborhoods influenced drug use. These methods, part of what the researchers label a larger "ethnoepidemiologic study," included the following:

1. Bringing intravenous drug users from a single neighborhood together to draw maps of the sites, people, and behaviors influencing their drug use. These maps, and the discussion they generated, helped researchers understand "the distances and pathways that intravenous drug users cover over the course of a day, as well as the type and spatial relationships of places of interest to [them]"(*Ibid.*, 2000:1050).
2. Observing and describing specific neighborhoods in the three study areas, including physical and social characteristics; locations of buildings, businesses, social agencies; zones of gang and police activity; and daily events recorded in newspapers. This allowed researchers to understand the specific character of neighborhoods and how they changed over time. For example, they found that heroin was sold in the morning in one neighborhood, whereas crack cocaine was sold in the late afternoon in another.
3. Having participants keep daily diaries of their drug-related and survival strategies helped researchers understand individuals' coping strategies, variations in their behavior over time, and contextual influences on these behaviors.
4. Accompanying drug users for half-day visits on their normal activities allowed researchers to experience how the drug users perceive and respond to the places they inhabited, how study participants interacted with a broad range of individuals, and how they managed the contingencies and unexpected events that occurred.
5. Accompanying a small subsample of individuals as they acquired syringes, and then using DNA tests to see whether the syringes had been previously used. This strategy showed what types of neighborhood sources were likely to distribute used versus sterile syringes. By putting this together with other information, researchers were able to estimate the likelihood that previously used syringes would be acquired in each of the target neighborhoods.
6. Interviewing and observing a subsample of participants as they injected and used drugs helped researchers appreciate the specific behaviors that might influence the risk of acquiring HIV or hepatitis from used needles and the social relationships among drug users.

The combination of these methods, rather than any one by itself, gave the research team a detailed picture of specific local contexts, variations, and insights about how to intervene to reduce risks in specific local settings. This is a good example of how contemporary researchers mix methods to unpack the complex processes by which intravenous drug use eventuates in HIV infection.

V.   Aspects of *Time*

A.   *Through What Social and Cultural Pathways Does Time Influence Health?*

Aspects of *time* can be as different as age, season, schedule, calendar time, or circadian rhythm. There are many obvious ways that time influences disease risk, most notably with respect to chronological age. Age influences to which diseases and injuries human bodies are susceptible. Infectious diseases such as chickenpox or measles predominantly attack the young, conferring a level of immunity that lowers the incidence among adults. Chronic diseases such as hypertension or type II diabetes and degenerative conditions such as osteoporosis attack primarily the old. Sexually transmitted viruses such as HIV are usually spread among those old enough to be having sex, unless transmitted at childbirth or neonatally through breast milk. But categorizing a few less-recognized influences of time on disease allows us to see new challenges for health research.

Anthropologists have long paid ethnographic attention to activity changes over time, cataloguing things such as seasonal rounds, ritual cycles, and cyclical migrations. Paradoxically, however, they have played a small role in connecting those time-centered activities to health outcomes. For example, if time allocation studies could be better linked to exposure to disease risk, anthropologists might have a powerful contribution to make to studies of time as a causal agent.

Whether time is conceived as moments between breaths, crops, moon phases, rotations of the earth, or more than nine billion cycles of a Cesium-133 atom, the perception and measurement of time is a culturally constructed activity. Humans have created and adapted to the relaxed timeline and schedule of hunter gatherers as well as the tense and scheduled stresses of the urban worker. How much time is spent exercising, and how much time a nervous system spends in an excited, catecholamine-flooded state both appear to influence risk of heart disease. How much time people make available for sick children seems to influence propensity to overmedicate with antibiotics and anti-hyperactivity medications. The instruction that pills be taken "three times a day with meals" shows that cultural assumptions about the timing and frequency of meals are brought to bear in regulating health-related behavior. The perception of

Table 3.6. *Recognition of malarial threat by season in Tanzania*

Percent of inhabitants who recognized a grave threat from:	Season		
	Rainy	Harvest	Cold
Fever from malaria	81%	50%	35%
Fever that does not respond to any treatment	76%	70%	60%

Source: Winch et al. 1994.

time, and the perception that time itself can exert pressure – be spent, wasted, or saved – has different effects on disease in different places.

Humans divide the world into units of time and associate certain activities and processes with those units to influence patterns of disease and death. Ideas about malaria transmission during locally perceived seasons helps influence whether some Tanzanians find it worthwhile to use preventive technologies – such as insecticide-impregnated bed nets – throughout the year. A study combining anthropology and epidemiology showed that time of year played a critical role in people's recognition of disease and their willingness to use bed nets (Winch et al. 1994). These researchers found that people accurately perceived fluctuations in the number of mosquitoes present at different times of the year but associated the risk of malaria with the concentration of mosquitoes, not realizing that the proportion of infectious mosquitoes increases as mosquitoes age and their numbers diminish. Residents did not realize that malaria could be transmitted year round. Most fevers were in fact caused by malaria, but in the low-mosquito season, people attributed fevers to causes other than malaria. They distinguished between types of fever not by symptoms but by the season in which they occurred (Table 3.6).

Along with the perceived etiology of fever, the willingness to use bed nets to prevent fever from malaria varied by season. During the "cold season," people were much less likely to perceive malaria as a threat, and therefore much less likely to use bed nets. In addition, if an epidemiologic study of malarial fever were to be undertaken in this site, the season of administration of a symptom-based survey would influence the measured prevalence of malarial fevers. Perceptions of time and its classification influence both willingness to adopt new preventive strategies and ability to accurately measure disease burden. Let us look at some additional examples.

OTHER CONNECTIONS BETWEEN TIME AND HEALTH

Anthropological insights could help to explain, expand, or refine some of the associations that epidemiologists have made between time and health. For example, there is some epidemiologic evidence that people are likelier to live up to or just beyond their birthdays than they are to die just before reaching them (Phillips et al. 1992). This link requires a symbolic attachment to a particular date and a mechanism whereby that attachment, expressed as a "will to live," a desire to avoid risky behavior, or another motivation, prompts or causes a physiological or behavioral response. Anthropologists might ask whether a similar trend in mortality happens in countries where individuals celebrate a saint's day rather than a birthday. Is mortality evenly distributed in places where people have other personally meaningful annual events to anticipate? Data are not available yet to answer these questions, but there is evidence of an uneven distribution of childbirth among Chinese in Hong Kong: relatively more births happen there during Dragon Years, which are considered lucky (Yip et al. 2002).

A second link between time and health is found in circadian rhythms and chronobiological research, showing, for example, the physiological reasons why heart attacks are more likely to take place in the morning than at other times (Portaluppi et al. 1999), why depression is linked to lower ambient light levels in winter (Magnusson 2000), or why women tend to menstruate at the new moon in areas without electricity (Law 1986). Research like this has led to suggestions that epidemiologists need to take time more seriously, reducing their present tendency to see health risk as evenly distributed across time. This rationale heightens the significance of the Tanzanian seasonality and malaria example: such studies raise questions about whether time measurements are taken for granted in many epidemiological research designs.

A more complex connection between time and health includes, in addition to seasonal events, connections between daily and weekly behaviors and health-related consequences. For example, more cardiac arrests in North America appear to take place on Monday (linked to the beginning of the work week) and in winter (linked to lower exercise punctuated with the heavy exertion of snow shoveling) (Gallerani et al. 1992, Peckova et al., 1999). Adolescent pregnancies cluster at the end of the school year in early summer (Petersen and Alexander 1992), and adolescent suicides are more frequent on Monday/Tuesday between afternoon and evening, after the school week has begun anew and when parental supervision is lower (Nakamura et al. 1994). All of these, of course, are predicated on the existence of a seven-day week, with a culturally defined day or days (Friday, Saturday, and/or Sunday) available for rest.

Unlike days, months, or years, the seven-day week has no astronomical referent.

These are good examples of links between time and person because they result from predictable and regular variations in behavior over different time periods. They also illustrate how culture influences disease: in this case, the cultural convention of a seven-day week and a five-day work week beginning Monday helps create a series of health-related patterns.

The time-sensitive behavior of professional caretakers also influences health: births in the United States are less likely to take place on weekends and holidays, no matter what the method of delivery. There are 14% fewer births on Saturday, and 21% fewer births on Sunday, than the average for weekdays (CDC 1993). Mortality rates are significantly higher for people with a few specific serious medical conditions admitted to hospitals on weekends compared with weekdays, presumably because of lower staffing levels (Bell and Redelmeier 2001). There is (debated) evidence that caesarean section rates increase before midnight or the weekend (CDC 1993, Fraser et al. 1987), and that the quality of medical care, or at least medical record-keeping, declines in July, when new hospital residents in the United States start their training (Shulkin 1995). There are undoubtedly many other seasonal and cyclical time and disease patterns awaiting discovery and investigation.

Less well-known and explored is the role time plays in how household members manage care. Medical anthropologists recently have begun to describe the ways that perceived time pressure, or "time famine," influences people's choice of medications, creating preferences for medications advertised as "fast-acting" or as specific for daytime or nighttime use (e.g., Vuckovic 1999). Time availability also influences women's ability to prepare nutritionally adequate foods for their children (Cosminsky et al. 1993). Other aspects of time famine were revealed in the 1950s, when household time allocation began to be studied in developing countries. In a classic 1955 study of impediments to water boiling in Peru, for example, poor women had trouble finding time in their busy day to build fires and boil water (Wellin 1955).

Finally, to bring us back to the link between culture, behavior, time, and health risk, there is a profoundly creative act of time manipulation in the United States every year: setting clocks one hour ahead early on the first Sunday in April brings more daylight during summer workdays. Clocks are returned to Standard Time early on the last Sunday in October. This creates its own inherent health risks: there are fewer fatal car crashes overall during Daylight Saving Time (Ferguson et al. 1995), and the number of fatal car crashes increases each year immediately after the switch back to Standard Time from Daylight Saving Time (Hicks, Davis and Hicks 1998). Thus the human decision to change clock time also changes mortality.

Time is the epidemiologic variable least explored by social scientists. I have described a few examples of the cultural patterning of time and of its effects on morbidity and mortality. Other fascinating examples await research attention. To be able to assess whether time exerts this influence on other kinds of disease categorization or behavior, Winch et al. (1994) argued that researchers should include the following steps in their research projects:

- Obtain a list of locally recognized diseases.
- Ask about causes, symptoms, treatments, and resources for those diseases.
- Ask if any diseases are more prevalent at specific times.
- Obtain a list of seasonal events/markers/indicators.
- Associate timing of events with months.
- Determine perceived relationships between events and diseases.

Similar exploratory strategies could be useful in many types of epidemiologic surveys in non-Western contexts. These types of anthropological methods of participant observation and analyses of meaning can play a larger role in exploring the effects of time on human health. In fact, although developed specifically with reference to understanding local categorizations of time, these steps also might be used to explore local perceptions of relationships between categories of person or place and disease.

VI.   Conclusion

Each topic reviewed in this chapter showed that some of the definitions and measures employed by health researchers regarding person, place, and time were culture-bound and therefore more arbitrary than the researchers would wish. Biomedical theories and cultural assumptions about the world pervade epidemiological studies, limiting the complexity, validity, and generalizability of epidemiologic results. To return to the notion of auxiliary measurement theories, what happens is that epidemiologists find statistical associations between variables as they have measured them, but they mistakenly conclude that these associations also exist between the (sometimes ill-defined) concepts underlying their measured variables. Evidence about stratification gets investigated and interpreted as evidence about racial differences; evidence about social context gets interpreted as individual difference; and evidence about human interpretation gets interpreted as natural fact. Early and extensive collaboration among epidemiologists and anthropologists and other social scientists using qualitative methods can increase conceptual clarity and analytic quality.

FOR FURTHER READING

Berkman L. F. and I. Kawachi, eds. 2000. *Social Epidemiology*. Oxford: Oxford University Press.

Centers for Disease Control and Prevention. 1993. Use of race and ethnicity in public health surveillance. Summary of the CDC/ATSDR workshop. *Morbidity and Mortality Weekly Report* 42(RR10):1–17.

Fitzpatrick K. and M. LaGory. 2000. *Unhealthy Places: The Ecology of Risk in the Urban Landscape*. New York: Routledge.

Gould S. J. 1981. *The Mismeasure of Man*. New York: Norton.

Mascie-Taylor C. G., ed. 1990. *Biosocial Aspects of Social Class*. Oxford: Oxford University Press.

4   Cultural Issues in Measurement and Bias

Q. What's the difference between an anthropologist and an epidemiologist?
A. The anthropologist thinks that the plural of anecdote is "data."

(Anonymous)

I.   Introduction

Anthropology and epidemiology are dedicated directly or indirectly to the study of human cultural practices and how those practices affect human health and disease. They must be fundamentally concerned with the theories that help guide and explain their discoveries as well as with the methods used to make those discoveries. Chapter 2 explained that these disciplines began with a fundamental concern for fieldwork, with the researchers always refining and adjusting how and why they collect information. Chapter 3 reviewed a few of the variables used to describe disease patterns, showing that new questions and concerns are raised when social scientists, particularly anthropologists, unpack the assumptions underlying such variables. This chapter pays more specific attention to the collection of data. I argue that data collection is built on a series of cultural conventions, not all of which facilitate valid measurement. Data collection is improved when those conventions are acknowledged and confronted.

The chapter-opening quote and Figure 4.1 show some of the cultural conventions around data collection. The quote portrays a standard critique of anthropology, namely that it studies too few people and mistakes mere anecdote for data. Figure 4.1 shows a standard kind of cartoon genre, the "public opinion poll." This one pokes fun at the pollsters and all the invisible interpretive errors that can take place between a household interview and a final monolithic summary statistic. Both jokes manifest some underlying discomforts about how we learn what we know. Why can't stories be understood and used as data? How can we know when snores are miscounted as presidential support?

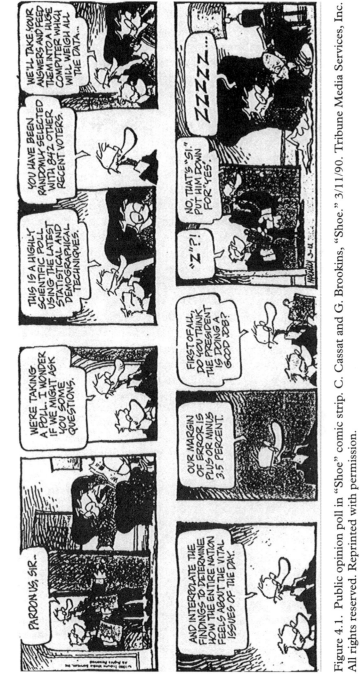

Figure 4.1. Public opinion poll in "Shoe" comic strip. C. Cassat and G. Brookins, "Shoe." 3/11/90. Tribune Media Services, Inc. All rights reserved. Reprinted with permission.

Three concepts are usually helpful in guiding discussions of the quality of data collection: *validity, reliability,* and *generalizability.* Although scientists define *validity* in many ways, the concept refers to correspondence between what one thinks one is measuring and what one is really measuring. *Reliability,* on the other hand, is the likelihood that a measure will repeatedly yield the same results. Reliability can be defined as similar results over time from multiple uses of the same test, or it can be defined as similar assessments reached by multiple observers. *Generalizability* refers to the possibility that a study's outcomes based on a sample also will apply to the broader group from which the sample is drawn.

Anthropologists do many things to avoid anecdote. They often seek to increase the accuracy of their methods by relying on *participant observation,* an approach to doing research that relies on long-term contact with a specific place and community. (See the description in the next section of how participant observation methods helped an anthropologist suggest culturally valid measures of infant mortality in Brazil.) Anthropologists commonly write fieldnotes to describe their daily experiences, but they also rely on guided observations, surveys, maps, and reviews of written records such as newspapers, parish records, or other archival data. Because participant observation emphasizes duration, breadth, and depth of contact, it increases validity at the expense of reliability and generalizability. That is, its strength is that it provides detailed information from many different kinds of sources about a particular place. Whether other observers would conclude the same things about that place, and whether that place is really like many other places, remains untested in most anthropological studies.

A.   Developing Ethnographically Sensitive Vital Statistics: Measuring Infant and Child Mortality in Brazil

Marilyn Nations has undertaken a series of innovative projects in Brazil combining anthropology and epidemiology. One of these studies sought to compare official infant mortality rates with popular (unofficial) meanings and experiences of infant death in the northeast region of Brazil, which has among the highest infant mortality rates in the world (Nations and Amaral 1991). The goals of this study were to measure death accurately and to correct any apparent errors in official population-level measures of infant and child mortality.

The investigators undertook 118 interviews with parents of dead or dying children in three poor rural communities. They observed healing ceremonies, child wakes, funerals, and burials. They learned that deaths in Brazil only get counted in official statistics when registered at government-authorized sites. But this process often necessitates multiple trips to a capital city and requires the services of a doctor to ascertain the cause of death. Parents are offered incentives to register a child's birth but disincentives to register a death: although registering a child's birth can lead to benefits such as milk and food supplements, school enrollment, voting, and health care, registering a child's death can incur penalties such as losing food supplements. Not surprisingly, births tend to be registered, but death registry is comparatively incomplete.

The anthropologists also studied the types of rituals involved in the dying process and the community members involved in those rituals. They used their data to develop a network of people who had inside knowledge of infant and child deaths: grave diggers, coffin makers, indigenous midwives, undertakers, priests, and the like. They then trained these people to detect and record infant and child deaths in one town, and they compared over 12 months the number of deaths detected by these "popular death reporters" to those officially registered and to those found in a census of all households with children under age five. Nine deaths of children under five were reported from all these sources put together: the popular reporters identified eight of them; the survey six, and the official registry only four. The sources assembled through anthropological fieldwork provided more accurate counts of infant and child deaths than the official registry or a household survey. The authors conclude that they have painted a picture of infant and child death that is more nuanced and valid than the cold and incomplete numbers provided by the state or national government.

And what do epidemiologists do to increase the accuracy of their measurements? They increase accuracy by relying on large random samples, standard (pretested) measurement scales, and tested survey questions. These methods improve reliability and generalizability, sometimes at the expense of validity. That is, epidemiologists focus on the likelihood that another researcher would find the same results that they did, and that the site under study is a good example of other sites like it. But because of unexamined assumptions and the popularity of particular types of variables at particular times, the validity and accuracy of epidemiologic measures may not always be just what epidemiologists intend them to be.

How do epidemiologists and anthropologists design research to obtain valid *and* reliable data? Epidemiologists divide their studies into *experimental* and *observational* designs. Experimental designs involve some type of purposive and measured intervention on the part of the researcher, whereas observational designs involve data collection without researcher intervention. Observational studies are called *descriptive* if they present the overall distribution of disease in a population, and *analytic* if they explain observed patterns in terms of proposed causal or etiologic factors. Observation and description also are essential parts of any anthropological study, but few anthropologists would describe intervention and experiment as appropriate objectives. By participating in the daily activities of a given group over time, anthropologists believe they come to understand what it means to be a member of that group. Anthropologists are thus likely to be able to compile more intimate and comprehensive pictures of daily life than could be obtained by a complete outsider.

One way to try to resolve some of the differences between epidemiological and anthropological forms of observation has been to create interview tools that combine descriptive narrative accounts of local concepts of illness with systematic coding and analysis. One such tool called the EMIC (Explanatory Model Interview Catalogue) was developed primarily to facilitate the study of local concepts of mental health (Weiss 2001). The EMIC uses a combination of open-ended and closed-ended questions, so that respondent categories unknown to a researcher can be uncovered and measured, but so also can measures of the frequency and causes of categories presented by researchers.

Anthropology and epidemiology are typically thought to involve dramatically different analytic processes, but there is actually a great deal of similarity between them. One traditional approach to anthropological analysis has been described as follows: the anthropologist commonly finds a behavior pattern in the multiple singular acts of particular individuals, then creates abstract roles and relationships from those patterns, and then seeks or proposes principles that can account for those roles and relationships (Nadel 1957). Epidemiologists also generalize about the behavior of individuals when they construct measures of exposure. They find disease patterns in data aggregated across multiple individuals, and they seek or propose principles that can account for those patterns. Anthropologists sometimes seem to forget that expanding from a unique individual utterance or action to a more general description of group context requires an act of descriptive abstraction. On the other hand, epidemiologists sometimes seem to forget that categorizing risk factors or choosing measures requires qualitative judgment. Thus descriptive abstraction occurs in both epidemiology and anthropology, although epidemiologists commonly seek and describe their abstracted patterns of disease using quantitative descriptions built from a statistical vocabulary, whereas anthropologists more often present their abstracted patterns of culture using qualitative descriptions built from an everyday vocabulary.

II.   Bias in Epidemiology and Its Anthropological Counterparts

Bias, or systematic error, is a critical concept in epidemiologic research. Bias is a threat to validity that cannot be resolved through additional analysis. Bias may inflate or minimize estimates, but if results are biased, then no amount of analysis will uncover the true values. Epidemiologists have classified as many as 35 different types of bias (Sackett 1979), but anthropologists reviewing the list will recognize many familiar research topics. For example, epidemiologists define "selection bias" as errors arising from systematic differences between people who are selected versus excluded from a study, and "referral filter bias" as the increasing concentration of rare and severe conditions as ill patients are referred from primary to secondary to tertiary care. Both of these can be related to what anthropologists and sociologists call "health-seeking behavior," namely the strategies people use to decide what ails them and how to cure their symptoms (Chrisman 1977). The next section compares epidemiologic and anthropologic models of the health care-seeking process.

A.   Selection Bias and the Ecology of Medical Care

In 1961 the *New England Journal of Medicine* published a diagram (Figure 4.2) that described the hierarchy of seeking medical attention in the United States. The diagram appropriately noted the differences between the rate of adults who reported illnesses or injuries in a month (750 per 1000 population) and the proportion who consulted a physician (250/1000), who were admitted to a hospital (9/1000), and who were referred to a university medical center (1/1000). But this analysis represented only the formal health system, which provides only a limited portion of all health care. The formal health-care system refers to government-sanctioned providers of care, almost always licensed practitioners such as doctors and nurses. Kerr White, the author of the diagram, himself noted later (1997:17) that it would be important to classify how the general public describes its illnesses and health-related concerns, and when and why it seeks care. This would include care from formal and informal or popular providers ranging from physicians to chiropractors to megavitamin therapists, and anthropologists would push beyond that to include care from parents, neighbors, priests, co-workers, and other sources of health-related advice and treatment.

Just such a revised picture of the use and sources of health care in the United States as a whole was created in 2001 (Green et al. 2001,

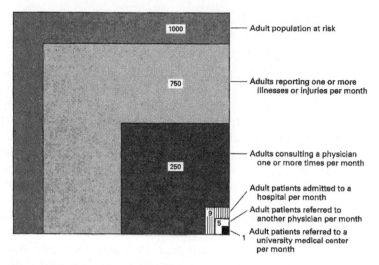

Figure 4.2. Monthly prevalence estimates of illness in the community and the roles of physicians, hospitals, and university medical centers in the provision of medical care (adults 16 years of age and over). From White et al. 1961:890. Copyright © 1961 Massachusetts Medical Society. All rights reserved.

see Figure 4.3). This analysis included both children and adults, and it described both biomedical and alternative sources of professional care. (It did not extend to nonprofessional care from sources such as neighbors, relatives, or co-workers.) The numbers were quite similar to the prior picture: 800 per 1000 reported symptoms in a month, 217 per 1000 visited a physician, 8 per 1000 were hospitalized, and fewer than 1 per 1000 were admitted to a university hospital. But, in addition, this analysis reported that 65 per 1000 visited alternative practitioners of various types, 34 per 1000 visited outpatient clinics or emergency departments, and 14 per 1000 received home health care. The proportion of patients in university hospitals and medical centers is very small in both analyses, although these are the patients about whom most medical literature is written.

Because so many studies of health conditions are undertaken in academic hospitals and medical centers, White and colleagues cautioned readers to be careful in generalizing from such studies to the general population. The article reminded readers that this distribution meant "serious questions can be raised about the nature of the average medical student's experience, and perhaps that of some of his clinical teachers, with the substantive problems of health and disease in the community"

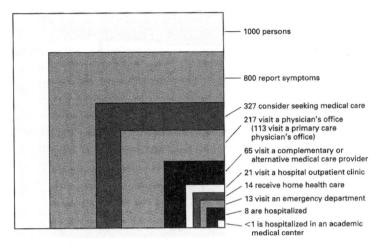

— 1000 persons

— 800 report symptoms

327 consider seeking medical care

217 visit a physician's office
(113 visit a primary care
physician's office)

65 visit a complementary or
alternative medical care provider

21 visit a hospital outpatient clinic

14 receive home health care

13 visit an emergency department

8 are hospitalized

<1 is hospitalized in an academic
medical center

Figure 4.3. Results of a reanalysis of the monthly prevalence of illness in the community and the roles of various sources of health care. Each box represents a subgroup of the largest box, which comprises 1000 persons. Data are for persons of all ages. From Green et al. 2001:2022. Copyright © 2001 Massachusetts Medical Society. All rights reserved.

(White et al. 1961:891). In other words, many doctors know a lot about disease but not as much about people. But it also is useful to consider how this diagram of the "ecology of care" would vary from place to place across the world in the number of symptoms recorded, the variety of sources of health care used, and the proportions of people using different systems of care. What is the "real" versus the reported number of illnesses and injuries in different countries? How large a proportion of the population is cared for by physicians versus traditional healers? What are the implications of this for where studies are undertaken? How should we interpret the results of published studies from academic medical centers in contexts where such centers treat only minuscule proportions of the population?

Some research groups already are beginning to combine anthropological and epidemiological methods to explore these types of questions. Take the case of Brazil, for example, which has the second highest rate of births by caesarean section among 12 Latin American countries. An interdisciplinary group in Brazil nested an exploratory ethnographic study within a larger epidemiological study to understand why so many women there sought unnecessary "C-sections" in hospitals (Béhague et al. 2002). The epidemiologic study of 5304 women looked at all who had given birth in hospitals in 1993; the ethnographic study selected 80 of these at random for more intensive interviewing and also interviewed 19 medical staff. The combination of these methods showed what the authors called an "interdependence" of biological, institutional, and social variables, in which rich women were more likely than poor women to receive C-sections, and poor women did things to pressure for C-sections such as arriving at hospital early in labor, seeking obstetricians known to do more C-sections, and requesting tests that might reveal a problem justifying the procedure (Béhague et al. 2002:945). Attempts to prevent or obtain relief for suffering have been described as health-seeking (or help-seeking) behavior (Chrisman 1977). These strategies of Brazilian women to obtain a desired C-section are exactly what anthropologists would label help-seeking behavior.

B.   Other Sources of Bias in Epidemiological Research

One potential bias in epidemiologic studies based on interview methods is "recall bias," defined by epidemiologists as "systematic differences in accuracy of memory." For example, in a case-control study where all people had the same exposure to potential cancer-causing chemicals, those people who have cancer (the *cases*) may try harder and recall more past exposure to chemicals than will those without cancer (the *controls*), thus biasing the study results toward an association between chemicals and cancer. Similarly, mothers of sick children may remember past events quite differently from mothers of healthy children. Recall can be influenced both by accuracy of memory and by changes in practice: those who have been diagnosed with a disease may change their behavior after diagnosis or treatment such that their recall of exposures is systematically more or less accurate than that of controls.

This type of change in self-perception and adaptation to a diagnosis has been studied more broadly in sociology as components of the "sick role" in adaptation to illness (e.g., Parsons 1975). Anthropologists use the term "explanatory models" to explain how people interpret their illnesses and present them to healers (Kleinman et al. 1978). Thus the social science literature on adaptation to and management of illness could serve as a useful resource for better understanding causes and severities of recall bias among different types of patients, and for different types of illnesses and disabilities.

The validity of recall assessments depends partly on how much time has elapsed since the event. Researchers have concluded that face-to-face interviews are the best way to assess uncomplicated clinical events and current or recent drug exposure, but medical records would be the best way to assess more complicated medical events and drug exposures that occurred years before (Horwitz and Yu 1985). The U.S. National Health Interview Survey (NHIS) researchers have conducted extensive research on how long after an event one can expect valid reporting: they have settled on a 14-day recall period for acute conditions and for health service use, 30 days for psychiatric symptoms, and 90 days for other chronic symptoms. Some conditions appear to make a larger impression and therefore last longer in memory: the NHIS asks about pain over the past 3 months, health activity limitations and hospitalizations over the past 12 months, and presence over a lifetime of certain chronic conditions such as hypertension, asthma, and cancer (National Center for Health Statistics 2001). The accuracy of reporting on health conditions is influenced partly by the period of recall. This is because low-frequency events are easier to forget and also because some events have greater impact on one's life and are easier to remember.

Studies of the accuracy of recall have been done with elderly populations in the West, comparing their accounts of youth and childhood with archival materials documenting their lives 50 years earlier (e.g., Berney and Blane 1997). These and other studies show that most people recall simple social and demographic information fairly accurately. Things such as occupation, years of employment, and residence seem to be accurately recalled by around 80% of respondents. Height and weight are recalled with a little less accuracy. Tobacco use is recalled more accurately, but food consumption is recalled quite inaccurately. So-called lifegrid methods can help create memory cues to social events like wars and strikes, family events like births, deaths, and marriages, and personal events like residence and occupational changes. Once these social, family, and personal events have been listed, the occurrence of other events can be filled in and located temporally near the listed events (Berney and Lane 1997). Methods such as these are commonly used to establish dates or other time references in studies carried out in rural environments, especially those where events and calendar time may not be linked as closely or recorded as carefully as they are in European and North American environments (Engle and Lumpkin 1992).

An additional source of bias in epidemiologic studies is nonresponse or nonparticipation bias, defined as "systematic differences in rates of participation among study subjects." Although two decades ago it was easy to reach potential respondents through phone surveys, today the proliferation of devices like answering machines, cell phones, caller ID services, multiple phone lines, and voice mail make it much more difficult for researchers to locate their desired respondents. Even when located, increasing proportions of people are refusing to participate in research studies.

This causes two problems: if those who respond are systematically different from those who do not, the representativeness and therefore generalizability of a study's results are greatly reduced. This problem arises, for example, in the current debate over the privacy of medical records. If people have the right to refuse to let their medical data be included in large-scale epidemiologic surveys, those surveys become increasingly less descriptive of the whole population. Population-wide calculations of cancer rates and cancer types may be one early casualty of the new emphasis on patient consent: in Great Britain the quality of data in tumor registries is threatened because people can now refuse to have their data included in the database (Helliwell 2001). This reduces the usefulness of the registry, which can no longer be considered a comprehensive source of data about cancer in the population. Similar concerns have been raised about how privacy rules influence epidemiologic research in the United States (e.g., Kulynych and Korn 2002).

The second problem of differential participation rates is of particular interest to *case-control* studies in epidemiology. Case-control studies take a group of people with a disease (cases) and compare their clinical history or behavior to a group without disease (controls), in an effort to learn what causes the disease. If participation rates in a study differ between cases and controls, this may bias results. When such differential nonparticipation is related to the exposure of interest, bias is inevitable. This happened in a study of cardiovascular risk: researchers were able to obtain some health records for those who did not take part in the study, and they learned that those who participated in the study had higher levels of risk but were healthier than nonparticipants (Austin et al. 1994). This would cause risk estimates from this study to be biased toward lower effects than would have been visible had data from the less healthy nonparticipants been included.

Although anthropologists have begun to study scientific research as a form of patterned cultural behavior, they and others have only just begun the ethnographic and interview research necessary to explain why study participation rates are declining or why people might decide not to participate in particular studies (see, e.g, Donovan et al. 2002). Of course, nonresponse is a challenge in *any* research study, including an anthropological one. A better understanding of how people perceive science and its measurement strategies would be useful to a broad range of health disciplines that collect data through interviews and record reviews.

Epidemiologists devote significant portions of their research to recognizing, labeling, and minimizing bias. Anthropologists use different terms and definitions of bias, and explore its causes, sometimes to minimize it but other times to explain it. This example of how different

disciplines treat bias in health studies points out that the same phenomena (e.g., incongruities between observed and reported behavior, or existence of varied pathways to health-care resources such as acupuncturists
and university hospitals) can be labeled, analyzed, and managed in quite
divergent ways.

III.   Data Collection as Social Exchange

The process of collecting data is often a process of social exchange. This
means that conveying information from one person to another is done
in exchange for desired goods or services (like money, future patient
referrals, or authorship on articles) or some sentiment (like pride, loyalty,
duty, or altruism). The social exchanges between a doctor and a patient
in a hospital, or an interviewer and a person in her home, can be quite
different from those involved in acquiring access to particular computer
databases or hospital record systems. But they are still social exchanges:
people with different backgrounds, interests, and motivations are coming
together to communicate across these differences. It is easy but perilous
for health scientists, particularly epidemiologists, to forget this.

The social exchanges between interviewers and their respondents resemble familiar everyday social interactions in some respects. Some people participate in surveys because they feel they need to. This motivation
is rapidly disappearing given informed consent and overload from market surveys: residents of the United States appear increasingly unwilling
to participate in person-to-person interviews of any sort (Atrostic et al.
1999). Some participate in interviews because they hope to get something
from it: the pleasure of having someone really listen to their opinions, the
sense that they are helping others learn or benefit from their knowledge
or condition, a way to fill up an otherwise dull day in a hospital or a
waiting room. No matter what their original motivation is, when they
participate in a survey, respondents react to the words and sentiments
of the interviewer. They may want to obscure or minimize characteristics or practices deemed sensitive, such as household income or personal
hygiene; others such as sexual practices or consumption of illicit substances may be minimized in some contexts and exaggerated in others.
Respondents may also overemphasize qualities or practices that are valued, like church attendance, time spent with family, or healthy behaviors
(Ross and Mirowsky 1984). At least where interviewing is a familiar form
of data collection, much of what takes place in an interview involves the
respondent's attempts to figure out what the "right answer" would be
and to calibrate how to make the interviewer see them in a particular
(positive) light.

Table 4.1. *Comparison: Knowledge/Attitude/Practice (KAP) Survey versus 24-hour recall versus observation among 247 families in Bangladesh*

	KAP vs. Observ.	24-h. vs. Observ.
	(# Discordant Assessments/# Comparisons between Methods) Percent	
Feces taken out of the home	21/58 36%	20/58 34%
Caretaker washes after defecating	37/95 39%	14/98 14%
Caretaker washes after touching feces	17/67 25%	14/60 23%

Source: Extracted from Tables 2 and 3 of Stanton et al. 1987:220.

A.   Are Interviews the Best Way to Measure Sensitive Behaviors? Asking about Hygiene Behaviors in Bangladesh

A study in rural Bangladesh was undertaken by an interdisciplinary group including a physician, epidemiologist, anthropologist, and statistician (Stanton et al. 1987). It was designed to compare the accuracy of observations, interviews, and 24-hour diaries as techniques to measure the presence of sensitive hygiene practices so that the appropriate (most effective) method could be chosen. Mothers' hygiene behaviors were observed and coded by researchers, and those same behaviors were assessed by personal interviews and recorded by mothers in diaries. Then specific behaviors were compared across methods. Table 4.1 summarizes some of the results.

The denominators in the results extracted show the total number of instances where two methods gave information about the same behavior, whereas the numerator shows the number of pairs for which the two methods gave different (discordant) results. Thus the first column, first row shows that for the behavior "feces taken out of the home" there were 58 instances where data about this behavior could be compared between interview and observation of mothers, and 21 of those comparisons had interviews that gave one assessment of a behavior while observations gave a different assessment. Thirty-six percent of the comparisons had discordant assessments. A discordant result is one where a mother was observed to take feces out of the home but did not report this at interview, or she was observed not to take feces out of the home but reported doing so at interview. These hygiene behaviors seem fairly difficult to record with any accuracy in an interview survey or guided recall of the past 24 hours, which suggests that they can only be measured accurately using observations. But note that the relative accuracy of methods varies across behavior: for "feces taken out of the home" the survey and 24-hour recall were each inaccurate about one third of the time when compared with observation. They were each inaccurate about one-quarter of the time for "caretaker washes after touching feces." But for "caretaker washes after defecating" the survey was inaccurate in almost 40% of comparisons, whereas the 24-hour recall was inaccurate in 14% of comparisons. So under some circumstances 24-hour recall might be an efficient alternative to observation for this last category of behavior.

To try to reduce the measurement error caused by changes in the way a question is asked or the context in which it is asked, researchers use a standardized interview format. But this type of standardization can interfere with the quality of the data collected. Two anthropologists analyzed a series of survey interviews videotaped for research purposes by the General Social Survey and the National Health Interview Survey researchers. They wrote that the interview is "a standardized procedure that relies on, but also suppresses, crucial elements of ordinary conversation" (Suchman and Jordan 1990). The presence of an interviewer and a respondent in a survey interview implies that a conversation between two people will take place, but many of the components of ordinary conversation are not allowed to take place at all. For example, the survey format gives the interviewer all control on speaking and topic, it standardizes the presentation and content of questions by prohibiting redesign of questions by the interviewer, it places specific limits on the forms answers can take, and it limits the interviewer's ability either to detect or to repair respondent misunderstandings. These analysts argue that the strategy of standardization in interviews "mistakes sameness of words for stability of meaning" (1990:233). They mean by this that the many strategies to standardize interviews can create bored and impatient respondents who censor their responses or fail to make themselves understood. They suggest that research designers rethink how interviewer and respondent work together during an interview, possibly by making interviews visually available to both parties, and definitely by encouraging interviewers to discuss meanings and to clarify their questions with respondents. One of the commentators adds that it might make sense for interviewers and respondents to complete a standardized interview or questionnaire following a lengthy conversation between them.

We face a paradox here: significant amounts of research time are spent trying to figure out how to increase response rates to interview requests.

For example, the following questions have received research attention in the United States in just the past few years: Do response rates go up if interviewers are the same sex and ethnicity as respondents? [Yes.] Do mail response rates go up if people are sent a token amount of money along with a questionnaire? [Yes, by as much as 15%.] Do they go up if an informational pamphlet about the study is sent to them along with the questionnaire? [No, not at all.] Does quality of communication with study participants influence their willingness to stay in a long-term follow-up study? [Yes, a great deal.] Does requesting biological specimens reduce people's willingness to participate? [Only a little.] Do people generally feel positive about participating in epidemiologic studies? [Yes, they feel they are adding to human knowledge and helping to prevent disease, although some have qualms about providing personal information.] Yet despite these efforts to increase respondent participation and understand motivations and causes of nonparticipation, the actual process of collecting the data still poses significant impediments to fluid and easy communication. This is one argument for using more ethnographic techniques to accompany standard interview practices.

B.   *Sensitivity of Topic and of Interviewer Influence on Respondent Accuracy: The World Fertility Survey in Nepal*

Two anthropologists wanted to understand whether women in rural Nepal responded differently to sensitive questions from an outside interviewer working for the World Fertility Survey than they did to sensitive questions from an ethnographer who had lived in their midst for one year (Stone and Campbell 1984). The anthropologists did the comparison, and they found that women did respond differently. The ethnographers concluded that the World Fertility Survey was "fully or partly unintelligible" to 80% of the respondents. For example, women interpreted a question about whether they had heard of abortion as a question about whether they themselves had had an abortion; they interpreted a question about whether they knew where to go to get family planning services as asking whether they themselves went to get those services there. The ethnographers concluded that women knew far more about family planning services than the survey suggested.

But not all information on the World Fertility Survey was equally sensitive, and a portion of the sensitive questions still yielded accurate answers: although contraception was sensitive and private and yielded inaccurate data, information about deaths of children and fertility history was sensitive but not private and yielded accurate information. This is attributable partly to the context of the World Fertility Survey interviews themselves: rather than being undertaken in a private area, both interviewer and respondent were surrounded by curious onlookers, and seemingly private events were held up to public scrutiny. It seems that the World Fertility Survey designers did not imagine that this social context would surround data collection, or they did not think it would be a hindrance. They could have done the work required to understand what the social context of the interview would be like. They also could have done the fieldwork required to understand which topics were likely to be sensitive and to yield inaccurate information. Their failure to do so resulted in statistically reasonable but invalid results.

It isn't only survey respondents who try to influence how data will appear: researchers also participate in social exchanges that influence their use of their data, and they also have beliefs about what constitutes a "correct" answer. Scientists developed the "double blind" strategy (which masks the identity of a study group both to participants and to the research team) because they learned that researchers also make both subtle and crude attempts to influence study outcomes (see Day and Altman 2000). The range of researcher influence goes from subtle and unconscious changes in question content or searching some hospital records more carefully than others to outright faking of lab reports and painting false colors on mouse fur. And it extends also to data analysis. One story I have heard in various versions concerns a statistician who wanted to show his collaborators the force of their prior expectations. He showed them a graph that displayed the results they supported and asked them to review why this happened. They readily did so. Then he confessed that he had mislabeled the graphs, and the data actually showed results opposite to their expectations. At this point a few of his collaborators refused to accept the results, even though they had supported the methods when those results appeared to agree with their expectations.

Data collectors in the field also influence data quality and accuracy. Here, too, the concept of data collection as social exchange can help explain systematic errors. Another bias identified by epidemiologists and other designers of surveys is called "interviewer bias," where specific types of interviewers differentially question and probe different types of respondents. A related bias in such exchanges is that of "reporting bias," where respondents are differentially willing to reveal sensitive information about themselves to different types of interviewers. For example, male interviewers produce less accurate information from respondents (both male and female) than do female interviewers, and "White" interviewers in the United States produce less accurate information about "non-Whites." The ideal interviewer for most household surveys in the

United States seems to be a middle-aged woman matched to respondents by ethnicity and primary language.

Sometimes data collectors seek to influence outcomes; other times they seek to maximize income while minimizing work. Survey researchers have to build in various cross-check and validation procedures to make sure that interviewers are not sitting under a tree or in a coffee shop making up data themselves. Though the following quote concerns surveys in developing countries, it is also potentially relevant for interviews in the United States:

We have devised the following descriptive definition: A rural Third World Survey is the careful collection, tabulation, and analysis of wild guesses, half-truths, and outright lies meticulously recorded by gullible outsiders during interviews with suspicious, intimidated, but outwardly compliant villagers. (Chen and Murray 1976:241)

Examples of social exchange to this point have been concerned primarily with exchanges between individuals rather than organizations. But the theme of exchange also is relevant to organizations and teams. It takes another form when researchers have to change their research designs to gain access to particular types of patients or types of research environments. This is especially true for epidemiological and social science researchers who do not provide patient care, since they must somehow obtain access to records or human respondents. Almost any social science researcher who has had to obtain permission to work with a group of patients can tell stories about how the study design changed in the process of negotiating or maintaining that access to patients. For example, DiGiacomo's efforts to participate in an epidemiological study of diagnostic delays in cancer were repeatedly frustrated by her colleagues (1999:438). Timmermans (1995) was forced to stop his observational study of resuscitation efforts in a hospital emergency room eight months early, and he also was compelled to invest considerable time in forming political alliances, exploring legal options and negotiating with the hospital's Institutional Review Board (IRB). The hospital IRB was promoting a particular vision of quality scientific research that did not respect qualitative data, and it protected the reputation of its parent institution and the medical profession more generally in the face of what it interpreted as unfounded criticism. And Casper's study of fetal surgery (1997) was shut down early when surgeons uncomfortable with her politics refused her further access to their patients. These are just a few examples of the ways that organizations influence the methods and findings of both staff and guest researchers.

IV.   Data Collection and the Challenges of Human Attention

Not all measurement error can be attributed to respondent or interviewer manipulation, or to what sociologist Erving Goffman aptly called
"the presentation of self in everyday life." Humans simply do not measure some things very well, and their memory of incidents, dates, and
faces often is exaggerated. The most public example of this problem can
be seen in the controversies over the accuracy of eyewitness identifica-
tions of criminals when these were later compared with DNA analyses. A
high proportion of people exonerated with DNA evidence were convicted
through faulty eyewitness testimony (Wells et al. 1998). Another example
is the major scandal over the "recovered memories" of supposed victims
of sex crimes and satanic abuse (see Pezdek and Banks 1996). In these
cases people were sometimes jailed 20 years after memories of childhood
crimes were remembered by their supposed victims. While not all the accusations were false, the majority apparently were, and their unmasking
served to reduce prior levels of confidence in the accuracy and truth of
memory.

But human weaknesses are not always as dramatic as false identification
of criminals or false memories of satanic rapists – they also extend to more
mundane memories of appointments and accidents, and to self-reported
health and functioning as well as that reported for other members of the
household. The following example shows that such differential reporting
extends even to something seemingly as unambiguous as male circumcision status.

*A.   Sensitivity of Topic, Understanding of Question, and Biomedical
versus Public Standards: Are You Circumcised?*

It seems improbable that something as obvious as circumcision status
could be subject to interpretation. Yet as part of a study of the relationship
of circumcision status to female cervical cancer, researchers in New York
decided to check whether self-report of circumcision was accurate. It
was not.

Male study participants and physician examiners agreed on circumcision status in only 65% of the comparisons (Table 4.2). Fully one-
quarter of participants stated they were not circumcised when physicians
thought they were, and 10% of participants said they were circumcised
when physicians thought they were not. Such differences could arise from
differing assessments between professionals and laypersons about how
much foreskin must be removed to warrant the label "circumcised." It
is possible, of course, that a high proportion of those men who reported

Table 4.2. *Circumcision status reported by patient and physician*

		Patient Self-report				
		Yes	%	No	%	Total
Medical exam	Yes	37	(19%)	47	(25%)	84
	No	19	(10%)	89	(46%)	108
	Total	56		136		192

Source: Lilienfeld and Graham 1958:715.

themselves as circumcised, despite lack of confirmation from medical exam, actually did undergo a religious or hospital-based circumcision, even if the physical evidence does not confirm this. It is also possible that those who reported not being circumcised, when physicians thought they were, had forgotten or did not know they had been subjected to the procedure, or simply did not know what the word meant.

This type of disagreement between sources illustrates the validity of diagnostic tests. If we were interested in knowing, for example, what percent of people who really were circumcised identified themselves as circumcised; we would be inquiring about the *sensitivity* of respondent self-report, that is, the percentage of people who really have a characteristic who are classified as having that characteristic. In this case, if we take medical exam as the "gold standard," then the sensitivity of respondent self-report is 37 out of 84, or 44%. That isn't very high if we want sensitive tests to identify cases correctly. The *specificity* of self-report refers to those who really do not have the characteristic and who are classified correctly. Here the specificity of self-report would be 89 out of 108, or 82%. Specificity is an important quality of screening tests designed to rule out particular conditions or to correctly identify those free from a sickness or condition.

One more layer of complexity should be added to this analysis: calling the medical exam the gold standard may be appropriate when circumcision is seen as an action with physical results, but not if we were evaluating it as a cultural category. In the case of cervical cancer, circumcision status matters because of the theory that risk comes from exposure to infection or other contamination from the foreskin. But meaning can be just as important as foreskin length for some health purposes. Under these circumstances circumcision status may be better assessed by self-report than physical exam. The question of whether physical exam or self-report is the best measurement tool here depends on the causal connections assumed in the research design. If circumcision status were being measured as an indicator of religiosity, for example, then respondent or parental report of participation in a ceremony might be a more appropriate measure.

Some surveys rely on one person to report the health status of other people in the household. Such people are called *proxy* reporters. When husbands are asked to be proxy reporters for their wives' reproductive histories, they do a poor job (Fikree et al. 1993). In the United States, proxy reporters tend to under-report disabilities in their households among persons under 65 and over-report them for persons over 65. Because there are so many more people under the age of 65 than over 65, researchers have concluded that interview surveys may underestimate the number of disabled people in the United States by more than 1.6 million (Todorov and Kirchner 2000).

Excessive reliance on spoken words in interviews can lead researchers to categorize respondents and measure behaviors incorrectly. Reliance on records of such interviews can cause similar errors. Some classes of information can be collected easily through interviews, but others must be obtained through more expensive and time-consuming methods of observation, diary, or other forms of interaction and collection. For this reason, ethnographic projects like those described earlier in this chapter are often useful precursors to interview-based data collection studies. They can help to predict which types of questions are likely to be sensitive and which methods can be used to obtain sensitive information accurately. To obtain valid and reliable results, some research topics will require the use of ethnographic methods to complement interview survey methods.

V.   Social and Cultural Aspects of Clinical Trials as a Form of Data Collection

Measurement techniques influence the quality and type of data collected. But the overall form and sequence of all the measurement techniques used in a study, the *design*, also is critical. Some epidemiologic designs, because of their complexity, cost, and popularity, are particularly subject to social and cultural influences. One particularly clear picture of this can be seen in the case of industrial sponsorship of clinical studies, especially clinical trials. In exchange for the extensive funds or specialized substances they need to perform their research, investigators have been asked to use research designs developed by sponsors or to sign contracts that give their sponsors the right to review and censor manuscript drafts in advance of publication. In the most egregious cases, this has resulted in companies denying researchers the right to publish papers that report their therapies as having detrimental, nonexistent, or slight therapeutic effects (Blumenthal et al. 1997). This type of agreement is a contractual form of social exchange because the company demands the right of first review of manuscripts in exchange for its financial or other support. Medical journal editors have become sufficiently concerned about this practice that they have tightened their requirements and requested more information from authors during the review process. (See, e.g., a summary of the concerns of 10 medical journal editors, in Davidoff et al. 2001.) Again, although this kind of agreement is most criticized for its limitations on publication, it also can have dramatic effects on the types of data collection techniques that epidemiologists and other researchers are allowed to use.

In a world of false starts, innovative but incorrect hunches, and abundant possible therapies, one should see many more published reports of failed studies than of successful ones. But journals show the reverse: many more studies are published that report significant results and successful trials. This raises yet another type of bias in epidemiology that has social and cultural overtones: one named "publication bias." Publication bias describes this propensity of researchers to submit and journals to publish primarily those studies that have positive (statistically significant) results. Researchers, journals, and the pharmaceutical companies that sponsor significant numbers of clinical trials focus on success, on innovation, and on promising leads more than they focus on failure to reject the null hypothesis. But if there is some tendency not to publish negative or inconclusive studies, then meta-analyses (which analyze data combined from multiple studies) will be biased toward positive reports. A study designed to assess the magnitude of this problem among research sponsored by pharmaceutical companies found a high frequency of duplicate publication, sometimes with no author name used in common across duplicate publications (Melander et al. 2003). It also found that research studies were three times more likely to be published if the results favored a new drug than if they did not, and that published studies tended to emphasize analyses most favorable to the experimental drug. They conclude that "for anyone who relies on published data alone to choose a specific drug, our results should be a cause for concern" (2003:1174).

Concern about publication bias is one force pushing researchers toward disseminating their results – especially negative ones – over the Internet. It is another instance of how new technology changes the research environment. But even if this technology does allow a broader range of statistically significant and nonsignificant results to be located and included in meta-analyses, how many people take the time to read the inconclusive studies, and how often do inconclusive or negative results make their way into the media?

Cultural and social considerations affect data collection about disease risks and health outcomes in myriad other, often subtle or unrecognized, ways. For example, interdisciplinary studies are currently more difficult to publish than discipline-specific ones, since the number of capable reviewers and interested journals is still relatively low. And getting a new journal listed in the large and frequently used electronic databases, such as MEDLINE/PubMed or Current Contents, is a long and difficult process. Some disciplinary journals face hurdles in proving their legitimacy to a biomedical audience, and so also do journals published outside of industrialized countries (Gibbs 1995, Trostle 2000).

Who is available for study, how accurately respondents reply to questions, how answers are categorized and presented – all these describe additional influences of culture and society on the construction and collection of data.

FOR FURTHER READING

Bernard H. R., ed. 1998. *Handbook of Methods in Cultural Anthropology*. Walnut Creek, CA: AltaMira Press.

Metcalf P. 2002. *They Lie, We Lie: Getting on with Anthropology*. London: Routledge.

Porter T. M. 1995. *Trust in Numbers: The Pursuit of Objectivity in Science and Public Life*. Princeton, NJ: Princeton University Press.

Sackett D. L. 1979. Bias in analytic research. *Journal of Chronic Diseases* 32:51–63.

Schensul J. J. and M. D. LeCompte, eds. 1999. *The Ethnographer's Toolkit*. Vol. 1–7. Walnut Creek, CA: AltaMira Press.

5   Anthropological Contributions
to the Study of Cholera

> Those with power were expected to take action against cholera. Those without power were the likely victims. Each had a choice of action, quarantine, cleansing, medical provision, prayer or just doing nothing on the one hand, and flight, anger, alarm, obedience to regulations, or just doing nothing on the other. Values emerged in choices between life and property, between work and safety, between charitable action and government agencies.
>
> (Morris 1976:18–19, on the 1832 cholera epidemic in Britain)

Outbreak investigations are a classic method in epidemiology; they have determined the causes of new epidemics such as Legionnaires' disease, Hanta virus, Ebola virus, SARS, and E. coli O157:H7. An outbreak investigation is designed primarily to identify the sources of unusual diseases or unusual numbers of cases of disease, as well as to prevent additional cases (Reingold 1998). The steps in an epidemiological outbreak investigation include finding cases, verifying diagnoses, and comparing rates with background expectations; interviewing both cases and controls about onset and exposure; establishing causes; and developing measures of control.

Disease outbreaks are almost always newsworthy and a topic of great public concern. The public reads many sensational tales of disease and heroism, real and imagined, with titles like *The Coming Plague, The Hot Zone, Outbreak, The Demon in the Freezer, The Andromeda Strain,* and *Plague Time.* But there are other, somewhat less thrilling, stories to be told about new pathogens. Outbreaks and the news they create also give the public a chance to see culture being created and transmitted because people invent behaviors and management strategies when they encounter new diseases. One small example of this occurred during the early days of the Ebola virus outbreak in Kikwit, Uganda. Villagers who were deathly afraid of contamination began to stop shaking hands and to start touching elbows in greeting, a gesture that became known as the "Kikwit handshake" (Chiahemen 1995). A newspaper photo in 2002 showed the captain of a cruise ship and a passenger greeting one another with a similar form of elbow touching. The ship was the site of a Norwalk virus outbreak that caused 524 people to develop severe diarrhea (Gettleman 2002). Shaking hands in greeting became briefly supplanted by touching elbows as a polite way to greet one another without passing the pathogen.

Anthropological outbreak investigations go beyond registering the development of new forms of salutation. In fact, an outbreak is an ideal moment for anthropologists and other social scientists to investigate disease: the insult is recent and noticeable, and people are still responding to it, revealing prejudices and assumptions about purity, pollution, and social stratification. When groups under pressure decide who deserves attention and care and who does not, or when groups choose which diseases merit rapid intervention, outbreaks show a society's fault lines. They also show how a society classifies its pathologies: is gun-related violence and death a public health or a criminal justice issue? Do we think about gun-related deaths differently if we call them an "epidemic"? How about 700 deaths in a Chicago heatwave in 1995? These were considered a "natural disaster" until a sociologist showed how lack of electricity and air conditioning, social isolation, and fear of opening windows in high-crime areas helped create the high mortality (Klinenberg 2002).

The steps in an anthropological outbreak investigation include identifying disease events worthy of study; collecting descriptions of an event; comparing those descriptions with people's expectations; and interviewing informants and collecting information from other sources about onset, exposure, help-seeking behavior, reactions, and interpretations of what is happening. Not all of these steps are needed in all investigations; some anthropological work might help identify disease event behaviors (or behavioral constraints) unseen by other investigators. This information then can be used to establish causes, describe or develop interventions, and analyze the social and cultural responses to interventions. Some anthropological outbreak investigations look like the discussions of constrained responses to the cholera epidemic described in the historical excerpt that opens this chapter. Others resemble contemporary journalistic accounts of such actions. And still others take a closer and more critical look at the categories and research methods developed to explain the epidemic.

This chapter relates one such anthropological outbreak investigation of cholera in Latin America in 1991, focusing on the epidemic's cultural, social, and political causes, as well as how professionals and laypersons reacted to it. Because cholera is one type of diarrheal disease, the chapter begins with the more general category. The first section shows that when ill health is seen as normal, this itself can influence health service use and disease epidemiology. Then the chapter examines the Latin American cholera epidemic, which was both unexpected and widespread, showing how an extraordinary illness can also influence health service use and epidemiology. I employ a model of natural history of disease that may be familiar to clinical scientists, but I then link it to a series of cultural and social influences that render the model anything but "natural." From this discussion emerges a sociocultural history of cholera that looks at how the outbreak influenced, and was influenced by, collective human attributes and actions.

I.   The Pervasiveness of Diarrhea: Implications for Epidemiology

The body has a relatively limited range of responses to a much broader range of diseases: fever, pain, vomiting, rash, seizures, difficulty breathing, and so forth. The term "diarrheal disease" describes one symptom that can be produced by a number of causes ranging from viruses to bacteria, parasites, malabsorption of lactose, or immune deficiencies. And diarrhea is no simple label. An extensive anthropological literature (e.g., Kendall 1990, Nichter 1993, Scrimshaw and Hurtado 1988, Weiss 1988) documents the broad variety of terms used to describe and categorize diarrheal diseases around the world and efforts to use these terms in prevention programs. Depending on the locale, caretakers pay attention to and categorize diarrhea using color and form of stools, age of the child, presence of a variety of supernatural causes, and other clues.

More than two and a half million children under the age of five succumb to diarrhea and dehydration each year (Kosek et al. 2003). Most cases of diarrhea are of short duration, although they may recur multiple times. Severe and extended bouts of diarrhea cause dehydration, which can, and does, kill with surprising speed. It is among the top two or three causes of infant and child mortality in most developing countries. Diarrhea largely attacks the young because weaned infants and children are more exposed to fecal contamination and less likely to have developed effective immune system responses. Epidemiologists commonly divide diarrhea into *acute* cases consisting of three or more loose watery stools in less than 24 hours, and *persistent* cases lasting for 14 days or more. Persistent diarrhea causes more than half of all deaths from diarrhea in many developing countries (Victora et al. 1993).

Although these facts about diarrhea present a fairly monolithic description, measurement of diarrhea is subject to a range of social and cultural influences. In the case of diarrheal diseases, accurate estimates of symptoms need to rely on maternal recall because most diarrheal diseases tend to occur among those too young to give accurate reports, and mothers are almost always the primary caretakers of sick family members. Reviews of research studies have determined that mothers tend to overstate the number of current or recent episodes of diarrhea slightly, whereas they dramatically understate the number of events that occurred more than two or three days in the past (Boerma et al. 1991). This has obvious implications for study design. To be most accurate, epidemiologic studies ideally should inquire about diarrheal events occurring no more than three days in the past. This means they must obtain information from many people in order to find recent cases of disease.

Patterns of health-service use make some epidemiologic classifications of diarrhea almost irrelevant to clinical intervention. For example, take the case of persistent diarrhea, defined epidemiologically as diarrhea lasting more than 14 days. As noted earlier, this is the primary cause of mortality from diarrhea in many countries. However, researchers in Peru learned that 85% of cases of persistent diarrhea could not have benefited from a standardized treatment offered by health-care providers because a large majority of children with diarrhea had in fact been seen by health providers within the first few days of onset but did not return even if their diarrhea lasted more than 14 days (Paredes et al. 1992). In this instance the epidemiologic definition bears little resemblance to what mothers care about. Anthropological studies of diarrhea have documented that mothers are frightened by their child's discomfort, burdened by the time needed to clean house and clothes, reluctant or unable to pay for expensive care, and eager to find some resolution (Bentley 1992). Additional visits to a health-care provider are simply too expensive, and mothers instead seek care from pharmacies, local healers, and neighbors. As a consequence, the opportunity to identify and treat persistent diarrhea can be lost.

Diagnosing acute diarrhea does not pose a challenge to most physicians, but treating it does. Although patients (or their mothers) simply want the diarrhea to stop, physicians are trained to prevent or treat the life-threatening dehydration that diarrhea causes. They could recommend oral rehydration solution (ORS), an inexpensive solution of water, salt, sugar, and potassium. But because the ORS formulation usually recommended by the World Health Organization does not halt the frequency or severity of diarrhea, dissatisfied patients sometimes demand stronger medicines that they think will offer immediate results (Kendall 1990). Physicians in many developing countries commonly prescribe expensive antibacterial and antidiarrheal medications rather than ORS to treat diarrhea, even though such medications are needed only in 10% of cases (Trostle 1996). In this example, doctors and patients often agree that the unpleasant symptoms of diarrhea warrant the more aggressive and expensive treatments, even when international health experts insist that ORS alone is sufficient to prevent most child mortality. While this conflict is described in greater detail in Chapter 6, here we need only acknowledge that the international standard for treating diarrhea involves asking doctors to stop prescribing the drugs they and their patients want, substituting instead a substance that does not give them the symptom relief they think they need. In this sense, physicians and patients alike are strongly influenced by the characteristics of the disease.

As mentioned earlier, diarrhea is divided into a large number of non-biomedical categories and is treated with diverse resources. Epidemiologists seeking accurate measures of the incidence or prevalence of diarrheal disease must take account of these popular categories or risk ignoring substantial proportions of perceived morbidity (Nations 1986). In some places diarrhea is taken as a normal sign of growth and development. So-called teething diarrhea, for example, is associated with tooth eruption because it often occurs at this stage of a child's physical development (Ene-Obong et al. 2000). Parents commonly do not link diarrhea to the changes in diet that occur when children's teeth emerge, nor with the increasing possibility of contamination associated with children's ability to move around on their own beginning at this age. The biomedical conception of diarrhea is not commonly understood among the populace of many developing countries. Many international epidemiologic studies have foundered when they assumed that survey respondents understood and shared the biomedical classifications of diarrhea used by the survey designers (Nations 1986, Yoder 1995). Because the condition is so common, people do not always seek treatment from professional or even biomedical caretakers, therefore surveys of diarrhea incidence or prevalence cannot be accurate if they are based only on patients who have sought care from official resources. And because local disease terminologies differ internationally from biomedical ones, and even in the United States (Talley et al. 1994), considerable care must be exercised both to understand how local groups define diarrhea and to develop accurate research designs to measure its incidence and prevalence.

II.   Cholera: The So-Called Natural History of a Diarrheal Disease

Cholera is a particularly virulent form of diarrheal disease caused by various biotypes of the bacterium *Vibrio cholera*. As opposed to persistent diarrhea, cholera is an acute infection, of rapid onset and short duration. To understand the cholera infection process in individuals, and to summarize that process for populations, epidemiologists commonly

Natural History of Disease

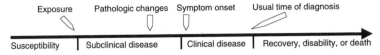

Figure 5.1. The natural history of disease. Redrawn from CDC 1992:43.

make reference to the "natural history" of disease. The model shown in Figure 5.1 comes from an epidemiology textbook published by the U.S. Centers for Disease Control and Prevention. It portrays a sequence familiar to most clinicians and epidemiologists. The pointers above the horizontal timeline mark events, moments critical to the progression of disease in a body. The vertical marks below the timeline mark different stages in the history of disease in individuals. Susceptible persons exposed to a disease may undergo pathologic changes (called subclinical disease); then may experience and perceive symptoms; obtain a diagnosis (clinical disease); and get assistance and recover, become disabled, or die.

Applying this natural history model to the case of cholera, individuals most susceptible to infection are those who have not previously been exposed to the *V. cholera*. In addition, O blood group or low stomach acidity caused by malnutrition makes certain individuals more susceptible to infection (Glass and Black 1992). People are usually exposed to *V. cholera* through drinking contaminated water, although some types of food may also carry the organism. Following ingestion in water or food, the *V. cholera* organism adheres to the small bowel wall and secretes a toxin. The toxin causes the intestinal cells to secrete water and electrolytes into the intestine in sudden and massive quantities (Rabbani and Greenough 1992). This is the onset of the pathologic changes caused by the organism.

Clinical and epidemiologic studies show that 30 to 50% of those infected with *V. cholera* never develop symptoms (Swerdlow et al. 1994, Tacket et al. 1995). For those who do, the most visible symptom caused by cholera is loss of body fluids through diarrhea and vomiting. Of those people who manifest symptoms, most have mild to moderate diarrhea and vomiting. In about 10% of cases, however, the loss of body liquids continues and becomes severe. This extensive fluid loss causes eyes to become sunken; skin to become hot, dry, and less elastic; and consciousness to become dulled. If the body fluids are not replaced through some form of external rehydration, death from cholera can occur within days. In very severe cases, death can arrive within 24 hours after the onset of symptoms (Rabbani and Greenough 1992).

Treatment of cholera includes oral rehydration or, in severe cases, intravenous rehydration, and administration of antibiotics. If rehydration is successful, full recovery from cholera can take place within a day. But while the human body is still infected, *V. cholera* is excreted in massive quantities. Further contamination can result from contact with cholera-laden sewer pipes, from latrines or sewage runoff from houses where people with cholera are living, or, more rarely, through direct contact with contaminated feces (e.g., in the process of changing bed linens or preparing a corpse for burial). During cholera epidemics, funerals themselves are one frequent source of additional infections, as are other public celebrations where people may drink water from a source they do not know is infected.

Following infection with cholera, people generally are immune to further infection from that same biotype. For this reason, children are more likely to contract cholera in endemic regions because adults have immunity from earlier exposure. When cholera is newly present, however, most severe diarrhea in adults is likely to be caused by the disease.

This so-called natural history of disease actually incorporates quite a few cultural and social elements that influence disease progression through time. Physical condition and economic hardship influence susceptibility. Work, diet, water source, poverty, activity patterns, and residence influence exposure to infectious agents. Once symptoms develop, they may be labeled and perceived differently, and brought to public attention at different levels of severity. There may be variation in who diagnoses the condition and in who offers help (a neighbor, respected elder, traditional healer, or doctor). Only some sick people come to the attention of official agencies of surveillance, and only some of those are counted. Sick people belonging to different social groups have correspondingly different levels of access to health services, and these health services provide varying levels of quality of care. Some medical care will be of sufficient quality and intensity to yield a successful resolution of the disease episode, but other care might make people sicker. All these sociocultural and contingent processes influence and help to produce the so-called natural stages this model describes.

Figure 5.1 described how disease progresses in an individual, and I used it to explore how social and cultural processes influence that progression. But one can also imagine a less familiar "sociocultural history" of disease, applicable to an entire population rather than just one individual. The sociologist Emile Durkheim, writing in the late nineteenth and early twentieth centuries, proposed that social systems need to be analyzed as such, not as collections of the grouped behavior of a set of individuals. Let us look at cholera as it progresses through the population at large.

III.   Cholera in Latin America: A Sociocultural History of Disease

Cholera has spread to large portions of the world seven times since the first decade of the nineteenth century, in pervasive epidemics called *pandemics*. During the present seventh pandemic two major types of cholera are circulating in the world, "Classic" and "El Tor," each with different levels of *virulence* (probability of infection given exposure). Cholera returned to Latin America in the form of the El Tor type in January 1991; the last previous epidemic on the South American continent had occurred in 1895. By the end of 1995, five years after the epidemic began in Peru, more than 1.3 million cases and 11,000 deaths had been reported in Latin America (Ackers et al. 1998). Cholera has become a major public health threat in the region and is now considered *endemic* there, meaning a self-sustaining epidemic. Capable of killing quickly and readily transmissible, cholera inspires understandable fear among individuals, national governments, and international health authorities. It signifies death and social disruption, potential export declines, reduced travel and tourism, and diversion of scarce health resources.

Cholera has both caused and symbolized similar social upheaval ever since its first identification as an epidemic disease in India in 1817. Diseases represent ideas about danger and risk and hope as well as malfunctioning physiology, and cholera is no exception. It menaced the British Empire early in the nineteenth century because it crossed all the important colonial boundaries of the time and caused them to be re-thought (Bewell 1999). It manifested the dangers of the tropics, the poor, and the unknown. It even showed the weakness of empire, since British commerce and troop movements themselves helped spread the disease. On the other hand, cholera also provided a convenient rationale for distancing the "otherness" of a dirty India from the sanitary regimes of colonial Europe (Prashad 1994). Instead of investing in fundamental infrastructure improvements to reduce the incidence of cholera and other diseases among local populations in India, local administrators attempted to separate "sanitary" foreign (colonial) neighborhoods from "filth-ridden" "native" ones (*Ibid.*).

A disease especially full of meaning and metaphor, cholera provides rich data for an anthropological analysis (see, e.g., Joralemon 1998 and Briggs and Mantini-Briggs 2003). It can be analyzed as "a well-adapted bacterium, as a symptom of societal collapse, or as a conspiracy against the poor" (Joralemon 1998:33). Reading cholera as metaphor as well as infection highlights the role of disease as an expression of society. As explained in the paragraphs that follow, it can be wielded to blame victims, offer a social critique, reposition identity, or change environments.

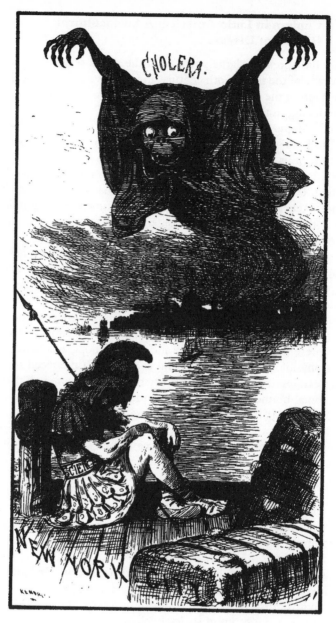

Figure 5.2. Cholera threatens New York City. *Life* magazine, 1883.

Sociocultural History of Disease

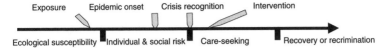

Figure 5.3. A sociocultural history of disease.

The cholera outbreak also provides us an opportunity to examine the distribution and use of a society's resources. When it returned to Latin America as a visitor from a prior century, it spread rapidly within poor urban neighborhoods and stigmatized populations. It was a grim reminder and reflection of the gross maldistribution of resources and limitations of modernity. This also was the case in the cholera epidemics of the nineteenth century, as shown in Figure 5.2 in a drawing from an 1883 *Life* magazine portraying cholera menacing New York City. The centurion guard representing the health establishment is asleep at the dock, and he is oblivious to the spectre looming up from across the water in London.

We can think of cholera as moving through groups of people over time instead of through an individual body. The model shown in Figure 5.3 of the *sociocultural* history of disease is applicable to an entire society. In this diagram, pointers above the horizontal timeline refer to events critical to the progression of disease in a population, whereas bars below the timeline refer to different stages of disease in populations. We can apply this model of the sociocultural history of disease to the case of cholera.

This population model requires that we consider how environments themselves influence susceptibility to disease. In an environment with a well-chlorinated water system and intact water and sewer pipes, the cholera agent meets a hostile reception and cannot spread. In another, where aging water systems allow cross contamination between leaking water and sewer pipes, cholera can flourish. This is why cholera was common in the southern United States in the middle of the nineteenth century, when open sewers ran down streets and buried water pipes had plenty of cracks.

The risk of disease in a group exposed to a pathogenic agent also is differentially distributed: even those with unhealthy individual habits may never contract a disease like cholera if they live in clean environments; those with healthy individual habits in polluted environments may still become sick. This is the stage of a sociocultural history of disease that I call individual and social risk. Risk is individual because motivations matter. Although people are influenced by history and context, some act to reduce their risk of contracting the disease by chlorinating their water, while others do not. Some with the disease choose to get care for it, others do not, and still others cannot. But risk is also social because some groups are marginalized to unhealthy environments where their likelihood of contracting cholera is systematically greater, and their ability to obtain adequate health care is systematically lower.

Diseases get labeled as epidemics once they surpass a certain threshold of known and accepted incidence. But governments usually do not assign scarce resources to epidemics until a problem becomes a crisis, and not all epidemics get labeled as crises. Some groups are important enough to society that the appearance of illness among them will be noted and attended to early. This happened, for example, during the epidemic of poliomyelitis among school-age children in the United States in the 1930s and 1940s, and in the early days of the anthrax attacks in the United States in 2001, when members of Congress who received contaminated letters got preventive treatment and decontamination before the postal workers who handled the mail. Among a group ignored, forgotten, or stigmatized, a disease may smolder for years before becoming labeled a crisis. This happened with AIDS among gay men in San Francisco, and it happens still with tuberculosis among the poor in many developing countries (Farmer 1999). As we shall see later in this chapter, this issue of who merits attention is particularly relevant for poor Latin Americans susceptible to cholera.

Populations eventually develop organized responses to crises, as well as specific interventions to reduce or eliminate the causes of the crises. These usually consist of a combination of education, treatment, and some related set of policy initiatives. In the case of cholera in Latin America, interventions included educational campaigns about water chlorination and handwashing, new legislation to control the food preparation practices of street vendors so that they would be less likely to transmit cholera, and repairs to sewage and water lines.

After an intervention the population either suffers significant losses and blames incompetent leaders or malevolent gods, or it recovers and celebrates the victory. Cholera created a rapid revolving door for Ministers of Health in Peru, where the 1991 epidemic started and was most virulent. Population losses there were consistently blamed on government incompetence. In Mexico, brushed gently by the epidemic, the Secretary of Health made cholera control a centerpiece of his long administration. Here population health did not suffer, and the Secretary served his full term.

Some authors have gone so far as to describe epidemics as forming a plot line with four Acts: Act One consists of progressive revelation of the disease, Act Two consists of agreement on an explanatory framework,

Act Three a sense of crisis that elicits action, and Act Four a drift toward closure (Lindenbaum 2001:367, citing Rosenberg 1992). This is another way to envision the types of changes that take place at the societal level in response to a new disease.

In the rest of this chapter I will continue this anthropological outbreak investigation of cholera in Latin America by asking three questions: first, why was Latin America a receptive environment for cholera's return? Second, what types of explanations were employed in the search for the causes of cholera, and what types of prevention programs and government responses did they engender? And finally, in what sense is this epidemic an expression of society?

A.   The Phase of Ecological Susceptibility: Why Did Cholera Return?

The cholera responsible for Latin America's outbreak is said by some to have been discharged from the bilges or ballast tanks of a freighter that had previously visited other infected cities, possibly in Bangladesh or China. This speculation may be true, but it just as clearly invokes a classic script by labeling the disease as a foreign invader from the Orient. Whatever its origin, the cholera *Vibrio* contaminated plankton off the coast of Peru. It grew well in water that was warmer than usual, perhaps due to global warming (Epstein 1992) or changes in the El Niño ocean current. Then the organism infected carriers such as fish, mollusks, and crustacea, and it was brought back by fishermen into Peruvian and Ecuadorian seaports. Unlike in the United States, where cholera has periodically visited oil platform workers in the Gulf of Mexico over the past decades but has never taken hold on the mainland (at least in the twentieth century), cholera in Latin America encountered a deteriorating public infrastructure conducive to its growth. This phase of cholera's development can be called "ecological susceptibility."

Human populations create environments hostile or conducive to different types of diarrheal disease burdens and organisms. Environments characterized by rapid urbanization, crowding, poor water supply, and poor sanitation tend to have massive fecal contamination and therefore rampant bacterial, viral, and protozoal pathogens causing diarrhea (Levine and Levine 1994). Environments characterized by better housing, less crowding, and good water and sanitation are sometimes also where commercial food production and rapid transportation predominate. In these environments there can be massive epidemics of diarrhea associated with food standardization and distribution. Levine and Levine (1994) characterize these as a developing world ecology versus an industrialized world ecology, but they point out that although these ecologies sometimes can be equated with national borders, there is variability within countries as well as between them. Developing countries have urban zones where the industrialized world ecology can be found, and industrialized countries have some environments with the attributes of the developing world ecology.

At the beginning of the cholera epidemic, most of Latin America could be characterized as having environments with high pathogen loads. Peru and Ecuador were in particularly perilous condition in the early 1990s. For example, a $5.5 million U.S. development project to install 420 water supply systems in Peru by the end of 1985 had completed only 10 and had started 20 by 1983 (USGAO 1983). Peruvian citizens were caught in a war between government soldiers and Shining Path guerrillas. One analyst has commented, "The processes leading to a cholera epidemic in Peru in early 1991 are linked to decades of chronic inflation that weaken a society's life-preserving systems" (Gall 1993:11). The country was suffering under hyperinflation that at one point raised prices by 7650% in one year, and this was accompanied by a decline in gross domestic product, reduction in per capita income, halving of public health expenditures, declining access to drinking water, and population growth in periurban slum communities (Gotuzzo et al. 1994).

Ecuador, Peru's neighbor to the north, was just beginning a series of structural adjustment programs to its economy imposed by the International Monetary Fund, following a decline in its oil revenues. New services were nonexistent or sporadic; existing services also were decaying. Without funds for extension or maintenance, the existing physical infrastructure of sewers and water pipes crumbled in many Latin American cities. In much of the region the institutional infrastructure of health-care institutions and systems of public health surveillance and control was under severe stress or was malfunctioning.

B.   *The Phase of Individual and Social Risk*

1.   MEASURES OF RISK
Even if the population of Lima, Peru, lives in an environment susceptible to infection by cholera, aspects of city life can either facilitate or inhibit the spread of cholera once the population is exposed. Lima has wealthy districts in the city center, but its rapid urbanization has largely been characterized by the growth of urban slums called *pueblos jóvenes* or "young towns," often the result of coordinated land invasions by hundreds of families. Areas of rock and sand are covered with shacks made of cardboard and scrap wood, and neighborhoods arise rapidly out of the desert. These settlements initially have no piped water, no sewage systems, and

no electrical service. Electricity is stolen from nearby power lines; water is purchased from tanker trucks. If tankers bring contaminated water the residents have no alternative.

Vulnerability of these neighborhoods to cholera is determined by both institutional and individual capabilities: on one hand, vast numbers of poor residents are given access only to polluted water; on the other hand, some of those poor residents boil or chlorinate their water to reduce their risk of infection. But epidemiologists tend to limit their definitions of "transmission pathways" to factors suggested in the individual "natural history" of disease model. These factors are primarily individual and behavioral, not social or political. The larger social and political causes of disease described in the previous sections do not tend to be perceived as relevant components in the chain of cholera transmission, as summarized in Table 5.1.

This table represents how researchers at the U.S. Centers for Disease Control and Prevention (CDC) described transmission mechanisms for cholera in studies conducted during the first few years of the Latin American epidemic. These transmission mechanisms are specific and are, in general, capable of being influenced through health-related interventions that emphasize proper behavior. With one possible exception, that of drinking untreated water from a municipal system, all the specified mechanisms are individual in nature and, at least in theory, subject to an individual's control.

But at about the same time that the CDC researchers published this comparison, a group of Latin American researchers (Gotuzzo et al. 1994:185) wrote that the "damaged socioeconomic system that causes extreme poverty" was the first of three principal causes of cholera in Peru. (The others they mentioned were the frequency of the O blood group in Peru and environmental factors such as increasing water temperatures of El Niño.) Cholera is a disease that primarily afflicts the poor because of their limited access to safe drinking water. But although this fact is known to all, poverty was not commonly investigated by U.S. researchers as a risk factor for cholera at the beginning of the Latin American epidemic. Ten years after the Latin American epidemic began, a CDC fact sheet on cholera stated that the risk group for cholera comprises "[p]ersons living in poverty in the developing world" and that "[e]pidemics [of cholera] are a marker for poverty and lack of basic sanitation" (CDC 2003). But these types of statements take poverty for granted. Poverty as a marker can be taken for granted, assumed impossible to change, and yet still used to justify quicker and shorter-term solutions. To call cholera a marker of poverty is not the same as calling poverty a target for a cholera intervention.

Table 5.1. *Mechanisms of transmission of epidemic cholera in Latin America, as determined in eight epidemiologic investigations, 1991–1993*

Transmission Mechanism	Peru (Trujillo)	Peru (Piura)	Peru (Iquitos)	Ecuador (Guayaquil)	El Salvador (rural)	Bolivia (rural)	Brazil (rural)	Guatemala (Guatemala City)
Waterborne								
Municipal water	+	+						
Surface water			+	+				
Putting hands in water vessel	+	+	+		+	+	+	
Foodborne								
Street vendors' foods		+						+
Street vendors' beverages		+		+				+
Street vendors' ice/ices		+						+
Leftover rice		+	+					+
Fruits/vegetables			+					
Seafood								
Uncooked				+				
Cooked				+	+			

Source: Tauxe et al. 1995:143.

Causal assumptions always focus and restrict attention. In this instance, looking at the causes of cholera as a set of specific individual behaviors focuses attention on behavioral interventions at the level of the individual rather than the population. The public health interventions in Latin America during the epidemic peak and afterward were targeted at the transmission mechanisms listed by the CDC in Table 5.1: they were consistently educational and personal, emphasizing behavioral change by individuals more than environmental or economic modifications by society. Ministries of Health spent their resources training physicians to treat cholera, and foreign governments donated supplies (antibiotics, intravenous rehydration solutions, laboratory supplies) and technical assistance for training and education.

I visited Peru in 1991, 1992, 1993, and 1995, and I lived in Ecuador with my family for six months in 1992 while I helped local scientists in the region develop applied research proposals to study cholera and diarrheal diseases. One popular billboard I saw all over the city of Quito during the epidemic read, "*Lavar las manos es amor en los tiempos del cólera*" or "Handwashing is love in the time of cholera," a play on the title of the popular novel by Gabriel García Márquez, *Love in the Time of Cholera*, published in 1985, shortly before the epidemic. By choosing this campaign slogan, the state emphasized not that social risk could be lowered through the provision of clean water and sewer repairs, but that personal risk could be lowered through handwashing. The implicit goals of government-sponsored cholera interventions were reduction of fear, case fatality rates, and political risks.

What types of data and analyses might be used to turn attention to institutional vulnerabilities instead of individual behaviors? A group of Ecuadorian epidemiologists (e.g., Breilh 1994) analyzed cholera as the distinct result of poverty rather than of risky behaviors undertaken by individuals. They used data from all municipalities in Ecuador to create an "index of deterioration" and found that it correlated with cholera incidence rates at the municipal level. Analyses like these take cholera as the outcome of a set of social and cultural processes, and they study those processes themselves in addition to studying the individual behaviors that bring people in contact with infectious agents. They thus see economics and politics as fundamental components of epidemiology. This approach is variously labeled the "political economy of health" or "critical medical anthropology" (Baer et al. 1997, Farmer 1993) in the United States, but in Latin America it is part of a strong school of social medicine (Morgan 1998).

Examining social and cultural causes of disease at the population level is part of the political economy of health. John McKinlay, a sociologist

Table 5.2. *Cumulative case fatality rates (%) for countries with more than 10,000 accumulated cholera cases, January 1, 1991, to July 15, 1995*

El Salvador	0.45
Peru	0.71
Brazil	1.07
Ecuador	1.14
Colombia	1.38
Guatemala	1.39
Mexico	1.42
Bolivia	1.98
Nicaragua	2.33

Source: Pan American Health Organization 1995.

and political economist, has used a much-quoted metaphor to refer to the difference between clinical and populational approaches to disease (McKinlay 1974). A group of health scientists is standing next to a river when drowning people begin floating by. The physicians jump in and save them one by one, while the public health practitioner begins to run away. "How can you abandon these people?" shout the physicians. The public health practitioner shouts back, "I'm going upstream to find out who is pushing them in." In this instance, Breilh and many other Latin American epidemiologists are asking society to refocus upstream on the causes of cholera, rather than (or in addition to) pulling people out one by one.

2.   THE DESCRIPTION AND USE OF THE CASE FATALITY RATE

Epidemiologic measurements themselves provide an example of institutional strengths and vulnerabilities with respect to cholera. In this time of rapid and ready transport and of available antibiotic and rehydration therapy for cholera, a percentage of deaths among cases (the "case fatality rate," or CFR) higher than 1.0% signals failures in the health system (Global Task Force on Cholera Control 1993). CFRs above 1% suggest that people are arriving at clinics too late in the clinical course or that professional staff lack training or supplies to manage cholera well. Among Latin American countries with more than 10,000 total cases (Table 5.2), official CFRs based on reported cases through 1995 ranged from 0.45% in El Salvador to 2.33% in Nicaragua. Counting such deaths is a political as well as a scientific activity because having a high CFR may mean paying political costs for failure. Governments therefore have an incentive to undercount cases, as the next section illustrates.

3.   COUNTING CHOLERA FATALITIES IN VENEZUELA

Political pressure on counting cholera fatalities was documented during the cholera epidemic in Venezuela. Charles Briggs, a U.S. anthropologist, and Clara Mantini-Briggs, a Venezuelan physician, were in coastal Venezuela for 15 months during 1994–1995 investigating cholera. Briggs had conducted fieldwork in the Orinoco Delta region of eastern Venezuela for almost 10 years. At the time of the epidemic in 1992, Mantini-Briggs was employed by the government as a physician and director of a rural and indigenous health program.

Briggs and Mantini-Briggs traveled across the Delta visiting many small communities and all the major population centers. They asked community leaders for details about each death associated with cholera symptoms between 1992 and 1993. Based on these interviews they estimated that about 500 individuals out of a total population of 40,000 in the region died in the outbreak. Most victims were classified by the government as indigenous Warao, although Briggs points out that ethnic identity is more fluid and less discrete than this label would suggest (Briggs and Mantini-Briggs 2003).

When cholera arrived in the Orinoco Delta, probably through infected mollusks, it flourished in a region long neglected by the State. The population already suffered from high rates of malnutrition and infant mortality, limited medical services, and difficult transportation. Although cholera had broken out in Peru more than a year earlier, the Venezuelan government had made few efforts to teach rural residents about cholera, and it had not distributed medicines or assigned the personnel that would be required if the epidemic were to reach the region (Briggs 1999).

According to Briggs, the government sent many resources to the region once the epidemic hit. But officials also "deflected blame away from government institutions and onto the cholera victims themselves" (1999:6). Cholera was depicted by the government and in the mass media as an indigenous ethnic problem limited to this group, whereas cases that occurred in mainstream society were rarely discussed. Individual behaviors such as food preparation and unsanitary hygiene, and cultural attributes such as food preferences and fatalism about death, were labeled the causes of the epidemic. The government and media neglected to mention the systematic national neglect of indigenous regions, the economic crisis and drop in oil revenues, or the poverty increases that had accompanied structural adjustment programs. The government worked to contain the political threat with short-term measures rather than long-term changes in health policies and infrastructural resources.

The impact of the epidemic was widespread and enduring. It could be seen in massive out-migration from the Delta to nearby areas, a diminution of power among traditional healers who were impotent to stop the epidemic, an increase in self-medication using prescription drugs, and an increase in stigma attached to membership in the Warao group. Briggs discovered this by studying not only the population "at risk" of contracting cholera but also the public health practitioners who responded to the epidemic and treated the sick.

The politics of counting cholera deaths were particularly obvious in Venezuela, where the government wanted to avoid the critiques and loss of prestige it would incur should CFRs climb much above the 1.0% that would indicate health system failures. In 1992, the country officially reported a national total of 2842 cholera cases and 68 deaths (a CFR of 2.4%) to the Pan American Health Organization. But Briggs reports that the regional epidemiologist and the regional office of health for the Delta counted 1701 cases and 49 deaths (CFR 2.8%) as of January 1993, then later reduced this to 823 cases and 12 deaths (CFR 1.5%) for all of 1992–1993. The regional epidemiologist faced national pressure to reduce the total by including only certain cases: "he was instructed to count only cases for which a laboratory confirmation was available – even though no laboratory [equipped to process cholera samples] was available in the state at the beginning of the epidemic and the tubes for taking samples were largely unavailable at the rural clinics in which most patients were treated" (Briggs 1999:20). This decision contravened international guidelines, which specifically state that "[o]nce the presence of cholera is confirmed [through laboratory tests], it is not necessary to examine specimens from all cases or contacts" (Global Task Force on Cholera Control 1993:37).

Even looking only at the government surveillance system, the politics of counting is clearly evident. But the 10-fold difference between the number of deaths estimated by Briggs and the number estimated by the Venezuelan government should create additional speculation about whose deaths get counted and why, and who gets blamed for being sick. This and other instances of data suppression are documented in Briggs and Mantini-Briggs (2003).

4.   THE MEANINGS OF CHOLERA FATALITY RATES

Differences between national and regional estimates of cholera case fatality rates are one illustration of what Julio Frenk and colleagues in Mexico have called an "epidemiologic polarization" (Frenk et al. 1991). The gap between wealthy and poor citizens is widening in most countries of the world, such that rich areas in poor countries have health profiles similar to those of industrialized countries, such as high rates of cancer and cardiovascular disease, whereas the poor suffer from parasitic and infectious diseases more characteristic of underdevelopment.

Counting deaths becomes especially political for national governments when the disparities between wealthy and impoverished regions are too glaring, and where national rates hide significant regional variation. The regional variation in Venezuela was seen in many other Latin American countries. In both Ecuador and Peru, some poorer provinces had CFRs more than twice as high over time as the national average. In Ecuador, Chimborazo, a poor highland province with a high proportion of Quechua-speaking indigenous groups, and Loja, a poor province in the south of the country, both often had CFRs far above the national average, as high as 8% during some outbreaks. Consistently higher CFRs also were seen in Peru, in Mariátegui, a poor indigenous region in the south, and the Nor Oriental del Marañon, a poor Amazon region. CFRs above the national average appeared to endure over time, even when the national average was far lower. For example, in 1991 the Epidemiologic Surveillance Office of the Peruvian Ministry of Health compared CFRs across different regions. Whereas the rate in the city of Lima was 0.25%, it was 0.65% elsewhere on the coast, 3.72% in the Amazon basin, and 4.07% in the Andes. Two-thirds of the cases were in urban areas, but the case fatality rate in rural areas was far higher than in urban areas (Gotuzzo et al. 1994:188). It could be argued that the government was providing poorer quality health services outside the cities, and especially poor care to the indigenous populations in the Andes and the Amazon. An average national measure of mortality masks, rather than reveals, this regional variation.

A complete analysis of variability over time in cholera rates at the municipal or provincial level would require collecting many data points over time, compensating for regions with small numbers, and ascertaining when high CFRs might represent the progress of the disease into new areas with low immunity. Consider what would happen if national progress were not assessed with a single average CFR but rather with a measure that would account for local variation. A CFR range might be one such measure, consisting of the difference between highest and lowest state or provincial CFR in any year. A coefficient of variation in provincial CFRs would be even better, since it would summarize the amount of data dispersion between individual provincial values and the mean value. Or one might compare provincial performance over time, looking to see how many provinces consistently had CFRs above the national mean, as a way of telling how an epidemic is managed by regional health systems. Researchers could focus added attention on the extent of a country's epidemiologic polarization, and whether this polarization is decreasing as the country learns how to respond to the epidemic or whether some regions continue to be systematically neglected over time. Expanding on the work done by Gotuzzo et al. (1994) and by researchers who studied the distribution of cholera across 32 Mexican states (Barroto and Martinez Piedra 2000), it would be interesting to divide entire Latin American countries into distinct ecological or resource zones rather than political ones, and then to combine case fatality rate data across countries, lumping regions together not according to national boundary but rather by ecology, altitude, resources, literacy rates, or other features. This has the potential to convey a more nuanced and accurate picture of the way cholera is distributed and managed. With data at sufficiently small levels of aggregation, one could even begin to look at variation within regions (see Oths 1998).

C.   *Care-Seeking: How Health Institutions and the Populace Responded to the Cholera Epidemic*

Cholera created an atmosphere of fear and menace in Latin America. Aside from the alarm about mortality itself, which was considerable, countries justifiably feared significant losses from declines in tourism and in agricultural exports. An economic study in 1993 estimated that cholera cost Peru almost half a billion dollars. Almost half of this estimate ($233 million) included future earnings of those who died, but losses from tourism alone were estimated at $147 million in 1991, exports lost $23 million that year, and health services spent an added $29 million to treat cholera cases. Income from new foreign sources of cholera assistance was calculated at $11 million for 1991 (Petrera and Montoya 1993).

Despite the enormity of the sanitary challenge, the study estimated that urban sanitation expenditures in Peru increased only $768,000 in 1991. This was at a time when the Pan American Health Organization was estimating that it would cost upward of $4 billion per year to bring water and sanitation standards to acceptable levels in Latin America. Although this was said to be impossibly high, it should be pointed out that the countries of Latin America spent $19.3 billion on military expenditures in 1992 and $21.9 billion in 1993 (SIPRI 2002). In 1995 Ecuador and Peru alone found the resources to fight a border war that cost each nation hundreds of millions of dollars, although no final totals have been released by the governments.

How did health institutions and personnel react to the epidemic? Cholera in Latin America was a disease of the past; it frightened health personnel who had never seen a case and never imagined that they would. When the epidemic first began, physicians afraid of contagion treated cholera patients with unnecessary precautions such as wearing gloves, surgical masks, and gowns. I had the opportunity to offer technical assistance to the Ecuadorian and Peruvian governments in the early days of the epidemic, and I helped bring a group of cholera experts from Bangladesh whose large international hospital, the International Centre for Diarrhoeal Disease Research, had treated upward of 1000 cholera patients a day. The Bangladeshis reported encountering significant levels of anxiety about cholera among clinical staff in Ecuador and Peru, so they spent many seminars just trying to reassure and educate the staff. At the beginning of their visit they created a stir simply by treating cholera patients without wearing masks and gowns.

Saving lives was the first priority of government, with cost and quality of care secondary. The CFRs presented earlier, or at least their aggregates at the national level, show that therapy was often successful in saving lives. Yet case management for cholera was far from optimal in most health institutions: the consensus of cholera experts is that many cases of cholera managed successfully in hospitals *never should have been admitted in the first place*. As mentioned earlier in this chapter, only about 10% of cholera patients are so sick that they need intravenous fluids, whereas the rest can be treated and released within a few hours or treated only with oral rehydration therapy. A study in Ecuador (Hermida et al. 1994) showed that almost half of hospitalized cholera patients could have been managed at ambulatory centers instead. More than one-third of patients were rehydrated with intravenous fluids only, whereas fewer than 10% required them. Another study in Ecuador estimated that about 45% of cholera treatment costs in a sample of hospitals exceeded WHO norms, with most of the excess caused by prolonged hospital stays, overuse of intravenous solution and antibiotics, and unnecessary laboratory tests and physical examinations (Creamer et al. 1999). In Ecuador, and elsewhere, patients sent home from hospitals with oral rehydration salts believed they had been mistreated. They described ORS as "nothing but a package of powder to mix with water." They demanded the more prestigious and powerful (and expensive and time-consuming) intravenous solution others had received.

Cholera also created perverse advantages. For example, the director of a national diarrheal disease control program in one Latin American country spoke ironically to me of "the blessed arrival of cholera." His program, and related activities in his Ministry of Health, received much more political attention, public prestige, and financial attention during the peak cholera years. Cholera treatment helped fill empty beds and employ underutilized laboratories at a time when bed occupancy was a critical component of future budget justifications. A Peruvian historian reported that "[t]he epidemic helped re-establish hospitals as sources of health care" (Cueto 1997:198). Hospital administrators found that the epidemic provided opportunities even as it brought danger and death. One hospital director reported to me that hospitalization of cholera patients was warranted because hospitals were sites of safety. He said he preferred to hold rehydrated patients overnight rather than discharging them at night to empty, dark, and dangerous streets. Patients sought hospitalization because absence from work could only be justified with a hospital discharge certificate or similar proof of severity of illness. As Cueto pointed out, for Peru, "The epidemic helped the population modify some of its expectations about health services. Free services hadn't existed for many years in the majority of hospitals, but this right returned with cholera and the population demanded to be attended in these establishments without any charge" (Cueto 1997:201). Thus budget processes, regulations about worker absence, and beliefs about treatment efficacy combined to create incentives for expensive hospitalization and intravenous treatment over cheaper outpatient therapy and oral treatment.

D.   Recovery or Recrimination?

At the end of García Márquez's book *Love in the Time of Cholera*, Florentino Ariza and Fermina Daza, elderly lovers, ask how they might continue their romantic boat trip without cargo, without passengers, without stops at any port. The captain responds:

> The only thing that would allow them to bypass all that was a case of cholera on board. The ship would be quarantined, it would hoist the yellow flag and sail in a state of emergency. Captain Samaritano had needed to do just that on several occasions.... Besides, many times in the history of the river the yellow plague flag had been flown in order to evade taxes, or to avoid picking up an undesirable passenger, or to elude inopportune inspections.... After all, everyone knew that the time of cholera had not ended despite all the joyful statistics from the health officials. (1988:342–343)

García Márquez captures the metaphoric power of disease, a phenomenon well-described by Susan Sontag in her books on cancer (1978) and AIDS (1988). Anthropologists are interested in the manipulation of disease metaphors both by governments and by individuals. I have described how government responses to cholera in Venezuela divided the populace into poor sick and rich healthy citizens. Another example of this type of analysis explored how government prevention messages divided Brazil metaphorically into cholera-infested and cholera-free zones, which mapped onto existing areas of poverty and wealth (Nations and Monte 1996). The residents of poor *favelas* resisted the government cholera control campaign, seeing it as a covert attempt "to contain cholera in slums and prevent its spread to wealthier neighborhoods" (*Ibid.*:1010). Nations and Monte described this seemingly inappropriate response of a mother who had tested positive for cholera: "Here we don't have cholera, no!... Somebody invented it! They are inventing it! And they are going to invent much more to come!... What do you think I am, some low-down stray mutt dog?" Residents responded to the prevention campaigns used by the local health department, which spoke of a "War Against Cholera," with strategies of denial, anger, humor, and ridicule of illness (*Ibid.*:1015). They interpreted government battles against the disease as a war against them. They were stigmatized by the disease, treated as sources of moral pollution in addition to infection. For these reasons they resented the government and rejected the campaigns. There are obvious parallels in this example to the reactions of marginal urban populations to the AIDS or drug-resistant tuberculosis epidemics.

IV.   Conclusion: Is Cholera a Signpost?

More than 150 years ago, in 1848, an epidemic of typhus was raging in Upper Silesia, part of what is now Poland. In Chapter 2, I mentioned Rudolf Virchow, the cellular pathologist and political progressive, who wrote at that time that "[e]pidemics are like sign-posts from which the statesman can read that [there is a national] disturbance... that not even careless politics can overlook" (Virchow 1848 [1985]). Medical anthropology focuses our attention on the interplay between disease as an outcome of ideas and practices, and disease as a cause of ideas and practices. As the sociologist Stephen Kunitz has put it, "Diseases do not simply happen to society; they are as well an expression of that society" (1994:142). Cholera is only one of many recent epidemics that have created and expressed social and cultural trauma. AIDS is an easily recognized example of this in the United States and many other countries; it was first identified by U.S. epidemiologists as a "gay" disease, and later as a Haitian one (Farmer 1993). The slow virus *kuru* in New Guinea brought accusations of sorcery and new mass attempts to expel evil spirits from villages (Lindenbaum 1979). Plague in India caused significant but unnecessary trade cutoffs by Islamic countries in the 1990s, at a cost of many hundreds of millions of dollars. The epidemic of SARS cost China, Hong Kong, and Taiwan billions of dollars in lost revenue in only the first two months. In each of these instances epidemics revealed particular rifts in society: poor versus rich, gay versus straight, sorcerers versus afflicted, Hindu versus Muslim, West versus East.

Anthropologists use a number of concepts that link culture to the understanding of epidemics, and these concepts are relevant to other disciplines as well. A holistic stance allows data on history, politics, and culture to be combined to understand why particular environments become receptive to disease insults at particular moments. Examining and critiquing individual and group risk allows categories of blame and types of intervention processes to be made more explicit and visible. Looking at how health systems change in response to new insults suggests new ways to evaluate health system performance. Revealing how governments use disease labels to create and perpetuate class and ethnic divisions is useful not only in evaluating and designing better health interventions but also in understanding how governments create and reinforce stratification. Finally, describing how a populace reacts to new interventions sheds light not only on the public health merits of the intervention but also on the social and cultural composition of that populace (Lindenboun 1979, Syme 1974). In some instances these insights can be used to improve interventions, in other instances these insights can provide an important external critique.

So the question remains: what does the cholera outbreak say about culture? Its reappearance in the Americas is a sign of systems in acute distress. Cholera mirrors the divisions of wealth and power within countries and between North America and South or Central America. It even reveals the immorality of emergency assistance: the U.S. Congress allocated $10 million in 1992 for cholera activities in Latin America, but it did not assign any special funds to a simultaneous cholera epidemic in Africa. According to WHO, the African epidemic killed almost 14,000 people among 155,000 cases reported in 1992, for a CFR of 9% (WHO 2000). Anthropological accounts of cholera probe and reveal deeply held ideas about risk and danger: the risk that the poor pose to the rich; that the sick pose to the healthy; that those who are suffering pose to those who are celebrating.

Although cholera transmission and treatment reveal particular components of human behavior and thought, other modern epidemics have their own stories to tell: AIDS, lung cancer, Mad Cow Disease, SARS, or any of dozens of other diseases also reveal how human groups are organized, ranked, managed, and sustained or exterminated over time. To explore this issue fully, and to learn what is unique and what general, would require more anthropological outbreak investigations (e.g., Briggs and Mantini-Briggs 2003, Farmer 1999, Guillemin 1999, Lindenbaum 1979).

Cholera is, of course, a disease particularly rich in metaphor, which is why García Márquez chose it for his novel. It is full of death and menace and spreads along social boundaries, but it also creates opportunities for people to offer a social critique, reposition their social identity, or manipulate their environment. These are some of the pathways through which disease becomes an expression of society. The main characters in *Love in the Time of Cholera* manipulate the disease to achieve a final transcendence. In the very last line of the novel, while the ship carries the elderly lovers offshore falsely flying the cholera flag, the captain asks, "'And how long do you think we can keep up this coming and going?' Florentino Ariza had kept his answer ready for fifty-three years, seven months, and eleven days and nights [since he had first laid eyes on his beloved]. 'Forever,' he said." (García Márquez 1989:348)

FOR FURTHER READING

Barua D. and W. B. Greenough III, eds. 1992. *Cholera.* New York: Plenum Medical Book Company.

Briggs C. L. and C. Mantini-Briggs. 2003. *Stories in Times of Cholera: The Transnational Circulation of Bacteria and Racial Stigmata in a Venezuelan Epidemic.* Berkeley: University of California Press.

Rosenberg C. E. 1987. *The Cholera Years: The United States in 1832, 1849, and 1866.* Chicago: University of Chicago Press.

Snow J. 1936 [1855]. *Snow on Cholera; Being a Reprint of Two Papers by John Snow.* 2nd. rev. edition. New York: Commonwealth Fund.

6   Anthropological and Epidemiological Collaboration to Help Communities Become Healthier

> The principle that health programs should "start with people as they are and the community as it is" applies both at home and abroad.... The problem is how to implement the principle. The real challenge is to discover just where particular groups of people stand; a willingness to meet them must be matched by a knowledge of the meeting place.
>
> (Paul 1955:476–7)

I.   Introduction

When I awake in foreign hotels late at night with jet lag, I sometimes turn on the television. This often is the best time to watch for official government messages about how to avoid malnutrition, AIDS, malaria, diarrhea, or a host of other modern plagues. Campaigns like these to increase health and reduce disease are an increasingly important part of public health work, although their appearance at 3 A.M. belies their importance relative to other shows and advertisements on television. Where do these messages come from, and why do they often appear when they are least likely to be seen?

Organized attempts to influence human thought, motivation, and behavior, and the environment in which that behavior takes place, are called "interventions" in today's public health vocabulary, and "intervention research" is its own domain. World AIDS Day (December 1) is designed to increase awareness of health concerns. Television campaigns to promote exercise, condom use, low-cholesterol diets, or mass immunizations are undertaken to increase behavior thought to prevent disease. Campaigns to reduce smoking or alcohol consumption aim to reduce behavior thought to promote disease. And work to design safer highways, automobiles, or consumer products is done to create healthy environments.

This chapter argues that anthropological methods and theories should play a more prominent role in community public health interventions for a host of reasons. Familiarity with community eases entrée and promotes better research and practice, whether it is to measure disease burden or begin a program to dispose of hazardous waste more justly and equitably. Ethnographic data about social interaction, relative social ranking, topic sensitivity, and similar themes are relevant to intervention designs just as they are to other types of public health research. This reflects the emphasis on "knowing where people stand" expressed in the chapter-opening quote from anthropologist Benjamin Paul. But as we have seen in prior chapters, anthropological analysis also reveals the social and cultural standpoint of intervention designers.

Public health interventions reflect prevailing evidence and prejudices about what problems can be influenced and what causes them in the first place. Chapter 2 showed that epidemiologists over time have produced many definitions of what constitutes a healthy or a risky life. The history of public health interventions provides a varied list of problems and proposed remedies, from removal of filth and noxious effluvia to immunization, elimination of poverty, and reduction of inequality. As epidemiologists increasingly have become focused on measuring health risks, they also increasingly have become involved in designing programs to reduce those risks – but in the process they have learned that knowledge of risks alone is rarely sufficient to design interventions that will achieve desired results.

When epidemiologists become involved in health interventions to change health practices for an entire community, they confront new and often unfamiliar challenges. Many a smoker or dieter could testify that there are dramatic differences between knowing what to do and being able to do it. And many an epidemiologist could testify that identifying behaviors that increase disease risk does not lead easily to effective programs to change those behaviors. Even the most captivating television campaign to convince people to exercise cannot have much impact at 3 A.M. Because anthropologists and other social scientists focus on links between individual and group behavior, and between knowledge and practice, they also can participate effectively in community health interventions.

Many of the examples described here are drawn from public health rather than anthropology. Public health has a long history of intervention design, whereas anthropology has an equally long history of intentional nonintervention. This is primarily because the discipline of anthropology takes differences across cultures as phenomena to be explained rather than changed. Anthropologists are trained to look for local rationales; they observe what they find rather than converting it into something more familiar. The anthropological subfield called "applied anthropology" has the longest, most detailed history of engagement in trying to create or manage social and cultural change. But much of the research of applied anthropologists historically was designed and sponsored by other disciplines or programs. Until relatively recently, health-related research in anthropology more often analyzed program failures than engaged in program design. For example, the anthropologist Philippe Bourgois has asked why there are so few prevention research projects in the areas of substance abuse and HIV/AIDS that combine quantitative and qualitative approaches (1999, 2002). This chapter therefore is intended not only to show intervention designers the value of anthropological knowledge and collaboration but also to help anthropologists better understand where and how they can participate in designing health interventions.

Researchers in public health have paid renewed attention to intervention design for communities and entire populations in the past few decades. This is partly a response to the new health challenges posed by chronic diseases like cancer, cardiovascular disease, and diabetes, mainly in more developed nations of the world. But they also have made this change because epidemiologic and experimental data from interventions show that it is more effective to intervene on an entire group than on high-risk individuals.

As part of this process of discovery, intervention designers have identified at least four levels of interventions, including education of individuals and groups, management changes in organized groups, legislative and policy decisions affecting society at large, and environmental changes manipulating physical space. The last three have together been labeled as "structural interventions," defined as "interventions that work by altering the context within which health is produced or reproduced... in the social, economic, and political environments that shape and constrain individual, community, and societal health outcomes" (Blankenship et al. 2000:S11). These intervention levels can be illustrated in thinking about how to reduce traffic fatalities. Physicians are educating drivers about the perils of drinking and driving; managers are changing work rules to promote carpooling or to vary commute hours; legislators are mandating the use of seatbelts, changing speed limits, and raising the drinking age; and engineers are designing cars and roads to reduce the overall likelihood of accidents and reduce the likelihood that any accidents will yield fatalities.

Yet these changes have been offset partially by citizens of the United States buying large numbers of huge automobiles (sport utility vehicles, or SUVs) known to be more likely to cause traffic fatalities than smaller, lighter cars. Asking what social, economic, and political environments shape this behavior would require us to cast a broader net. Which American values help citizens choose to purchase large SUVs? Are they simply trying to protect themselves from other drivers in large SUVs? Why do U.S. tax codes promote faster write-offs for large vehicles, and why do vehicle emissions policies promote trucks? Do gasoline pricing and the politics of oil exploration promote high fuel consumption? If so, should SUV sales simply be explained as "satisfying the desires of the consumer"? Thinking about structural interventions helps us to create more comprehensive explanations of the causes of illness and premature death.

Educational, managerial, and legislative interventions are most effective when they are mutually reinforcing, creating new cultural expectations. For example, the struggle to reduce cigarette smoking in the United States was ineffective when it relied primarily on educational messages about the health effects of tobacco use. It became more effective when the availability of cigarettes to minors was limited by reducing the number and changing the locations of cigarette vending machines and by making sales to minors illegal, when smoke-free zones were created, and when cigarette excise taxes were raised, making smoking more expensive. But it became truly powerful for some groups when these interventions were reinforced by cultural changes labeling smoking dirty, uncool, and obnoxious rather than sophisticated and enticing. Thus it is important to discuss the cultural context of each of these intervention levels and to show how anthropologists have contributed to their design and implementation.

A.   Educational Interventions

Educational interventions in public health are generally based on theories about the importance of information to health behavior. Knowledge is obviously important in changing health-related practices because it works on so many levels at once. People can act purposively only when they know what to do; they are more motivated to act if they know they are personally menaced; in general they prefer truth to falsehood. All of these dimensions can be influenced by education, and by the knowledge that education seeks to produce. Education for literacy, especially literacy for girls, is well-documented to influence many indicators of health and well-being (World Bank 1999). But anthropologists and other social scientists have raised many doubts regarding the assumption that education about specific health issues is a critical intervention by itself (Hahn 1999, Kendall 1989, Paredes et al. 1996).

Knowledge about health and disease, while important, is not always necessary and sufficient to bring about change. A college student may know what smoke does to her lungs, but her addiction and peer group pressure and habit will act as strong disincentives for her to act as her knowledge would direct. In fact, smoking among college students is increasing in the United States (Wechsler et al. 1998). College students, like many other people, do not always think about the actions they undertake, and, even when they do, their knowledge of what to do may not allow them to overcome barriers like nicotine addiction or incentives like peer pressure.

Another assumption behind most education interventions is that knowledge flows from the top to the bottom of social hierarchies, and from experts to lay people. According to this position, if people act in ways that professionals deem unhealthy, they must do so from ignorance. Knowledge provided by professionals will bring about proper behavior. But all groups have specific knowledge, and they use this knowledge to guide and justify their behaviors. A metaphor called "the fallacy of the empty vessel" was used to highlight this problem in a 1963 review of medical anthropology (Polgar 1963). Stephen Polgar, a colleague of John Cassel's at the University of North Carolina (see Chapter 2), wrote that people are not empty vessels waiting to be filled with the latest and most advanced knowledge. They work out their own accommodations to local health constraints over time, and their accommodations to local circumstance form coherent systems of belief and behavior. Information in health campaigns often fails to convince an audience that already holds competing understandings and beliefs.

The concept of "local knowledge" has long been of interest to anthropologists. This phrase emphasizes that knowledge has many different definitions, and that local systems of knowledge often compete with more widespread, dominant, national and international systems of knowledge. For example, local classifications and treatments of disease can conflict with biomedical explanations and pharmaceutical remedies for the same ailments. Knowledge about health moves in many directions, and educational campaigns about health must take pre-existing and competing knowledge into account.

Campaigns to educate poor urban Peruvians about the need to boil water are an example of what can happen when educational interventions fail to take local knowledge and context into account. Two research studies at very different points in time looked at why public health interventions failed to change rates of water boiling in Peru. The first, by anthropologist Edward Wellin in 1953, concluded that decisions to boil or not to boil water were made for many diverse reasons, with education playing only a minor role (Wellin 1955:100ff). Reasons for boiling ranged from feeling sickly to rejecting local values about cleanliness to wanting to satisfy the outreach worker. Reasons for not boiling ranged from not having time to not accepting new health values. Wellin emphasized that "it is not enough that action workers know the items of custom that characterize the community's way of life; they must also understand how these customs are linked with one another" (1955:100–101). An interdisciplinary study in Peru some four decades later found similar linked processes still impeding water boiling: this time researchers concluded that residents did not have enough water to begin with, but they also lacked the resources to pay for the extra fuel and often did not even possess the extra pot needed to store the boiled water safely during the day (Gilman et al. 1993). The fact that two studies separated by four decades point to similar impediments to water boiling further shows that researchers' knowledge is not sufficient to create effective interventions.

Many public health interventions today are designed to increase some particular behavior like water boiling, smoking, or condom use in a specified population like rural mothers, adolescent girls, or clients of sex workers. Epidemiologists involved in these types of interventions sometimes appear to assume that the design of effective interventions depends most heavily on accurately identifying risk factors. But communication theorist Robert Hornik, who was involved in community studies to reduce heart disease, has argued that data on risk factors themselves are insufficient to design effective intervention campaigns. Instead, Hornik contends, one needs to know the risks for the risk factors in order to design interventions that will influence those underlying causes (Hornik 1990: personal communication). For example, knowledge that saturated fats are a strong dietary risk factor for heart disease must be combined with knowledge about why people consume saturated fats.

This also has been called the difference between proximate and ultimate causes. An epidemiologic study of the causes of diarrheal disease may show that drinking contaminated water is a major risk factor or the proximate cause of disease. But an intervention to increase water boiling can only succeed when people have the needed resources such as water, pots, time, and fuel. Lack of resources, rather than failure to boil water, is the ultimate cause of this disease. This is an epidemiological restatement of Wellin's point: knowing "items of custom" is not the same as knowing how customs are linked, nor is it the same as knowing whether new behaviors are feasible in an old context. Knowing which behaviors pose greatest risk is not the same as knowing whether behaviors are interdependent, or whether they can be modified. In fact, it could be argued that if knowledge is an attribute of populations, the "knowing risks for risks" rationale should cause intervention designers to study the underlying sources of local knowledge and ignorance at the population level.

Educational interventions tend to ignore history, politics, and environment. Much as peer group pressure or addiction can diminish knowledge-based motivation to change behavior, so also can government neglect, poverty, and powerlessness inhibit health-related change, as we have seen in the water-boiling example. Political and social ideologies are a relevant part of that environment. Dramatic new state-level initiatives are difficult to design and implement in sites where health responsibilities have long been thought to reside in individuals. Take the case of medication use. Almost all countries in the world place extensive limits on what is called "direct to consumer" advertising of pharmaceuticals, and almost all have rejected attempts to weaken these limits. They reason that drug companies will use advertising to place extra pressure on consumers to request new and expensive drugs without knowledge of their efficacy. But in the United States many forces are arrayed against promoting more rational use of medications by consumers and prescribers. Rhetoric about free choice, freedom to advertise, consumer power, and physician control are all marshaled in support of limited governmental regulation and control of prescribing. Education about proper prescribing takes place within a context that limits the effectiveness of that education.

Or return to anti-smoking campaigns. Public health campaigns in the United States focused for decades on "getting the message out" that smoking caused lung cancer, heart disease, stroke, miscarriages, and fetal defects. But practically any U.S. citizen can remember (and still see) the tiny print size and poor location of these mandated educational messages on cigarette packets and advertisements in newspapers and on billboards. Knowledge that smoking kills when used as directed is not sufficient to prevent adolescents from starting to smoke (Romer and Jamieson 2001). The increase in smoking among U.S. college students shows this all too well. Creative advertisers put favorable images of smoking on race cars, golf games, cartoon characters, free samples, clothing, billboards, and sports arenas, and in movies, videos, and magazines, and these images create a climate that encourages smoking despite the known health risks. Tobacco companies have complained bitterly about, and taken legal action against, aggressive anti-smoking media campaigns targeted at U.S. adolescents (see www.americanlegacy.org). Anti-smoking ads are effective not because they offer new education about risk but rather because they counter favorable images of mountains and cowboys with equal (or more powerful) unfavorable images of body bags and overflowing ashtrays.

Information and education themselves are rarely sufficient to prompt change. This point opens another area where anthropological knowledge and training are relevant to intervention design. Some of the "risk factors for risk factors" or "ultimate determinants" of behavior are functions of motivation and perceived risk – domains of meaning and perception where anthropologists often practice their craft. Anthropological studies of behavior and of the perceived risks and benefits of changing behavior can reveal the complex motivations for action and the types of incentives that will inhibit or facilitate behavior change.

A focus on educational interventions has a built-in bias toward seeing health problems as functions of individual irresponsibility on one hand, or cultural backwardness or maladaptation on the other. After all, if it is easy to blame people for being ignorant; it is easier to blame them, or their culture, when they continue to damage their health by doing things they (or others) know they should not. This type of focus on culture has a number of pitfalls. Paul Farmer, an anthropologist and clinician at Harvard, argues that structural violence is obscured by labeling health inequalities as products of cultural difference, and that this minimizes the roles of poverty and inequality and exaggerates the extent of patient control (1999:47–50). Directing interventions toward individuals rather than toward organizations or politics is itself a political statement of support for the status quo.

B.   Managerial and Administrative Interventions

A second type of intervention involves the managerial or administrative level of organizations. Such interventions often take place in hospitals and clinics, although they also could take place at any worksite or other organized activity with identifiable leadership. They consist of changes in work practices or management policies or other rules designed to guide behavior at a particular site. Some examples from health services include modifications to rules about record-keeping, second opinions, or case audits, as well as decisions to implement in-service training or other continuing-education activities for an entire staff. Managerial and administrative interventions also have been used by owners of brothels to increase condom use (Hanenberg and Rojanapithayakom 1996), schools to improve student nutrition or teacher performance in health classes (Downey et al. 1988), cities to reduce stress and absenteeism among bus drivers (Kompier et al. 2000), and businesses to reduce violence among employees (Loomis et al. 2002).

Studies of service-based risk factors often contribute to managerial and administrative interventions. For example, epidemiologic studies showed that hospital provision of infant formula to new mothers was one significant impediment to early and successful initiation of breastfeeding. Hospitals were asked to change whether formula was available, to whom, and in what quantities. (These changes also were pushed by a well-organized boycott of infant formula producers, which will be described shortly.) "Baby-friendly" interventions, developed by UNICEF and WHO, broadened managerial interventions in hospitals to promote breastfeeding: they disseminated written policies that promote breastfeeding, trained staff in their implementation, allowed mothers to "room in" with their babies, and encouraged breastfeeding on demand. Managerial interventions can profit from extensive ethnographic knowledge about staff motivations and incentive systems. Efforts to reduce inappropriate distribution of baby formula by nurses in China benefited by having anthropologists, who used observations and open-ended interviewing, identify what sources of information new mothers deemed authoritative and what roles industrial representatives or free samples played (see, e.g., Gottschang 2000).

Managerial interventions, by definition, are used in workplaces. They are especially important in the realm of occupational and environmental health, where researchers seek ways to organize worksites to expose workers to fewer hazards. Yet anthropologists rarely study the relationships between worker organization and worksite health (see Janes and Ames 1992 for an exception). They are not the only ones neglecting this area: new ways to organize production (e.g., total quality management, modular manufacturing) have not yet been well evaluated for their impact on occupational injuries or job stress (Landsbergis et al. 1999).

These types of interventions may be completely ineffective if they are not preceded by extensive studies of how administrative policies and management practices influence existing behavior. The anthropologist Judith Justice provided an important example of a managerial intervention in Nepal when she described the failure of a program to send assistant nurse-midwives to rural areas in Nepal (Justice 1999). The program, enacted largely as a result of international pressure, paid insufficient attention to the political context and culture. Local concerns, like role expectations for single women in rural health posts and the questionable authority of young unmarried and childless women trying to work as midwives, ultimately defeated it. The ill-fated effort also failed to consider the professional concerns of assistant nurse-midwives, who expected to improve their job status and security by living in urban areas.

Interventions to change managerial or administrative practices should not be undertaken or understood as actions separate from their institutional and public context. When institutions change management practices they also make public statements about their values and goals, and their internal policies usually reflect outside pressures and broad concerns. These policies help to create ongoing roles by individuals inside organizations, and the resulting organizational culture is maintained through training, incentive systems, habit, and preference. To be truly effective, managerial interventions must be part of a changing organizational culture.

C. *Legislative Interventions*

Legislative interventions often cover large audiences and usually carry explicit premiums (e.g., tax incentives) or penalties (e.g., fines or jail terms). To revisit the example of breastfeeding, legislative interventions designed to increase breastfeeding could repeal laws that prohibit women from breastfeeding in public, pass legislation that limits sales of infant formula, increase taxes on formula, outlaw distribution of free formula in hospitals, or broaden parental leave policies so that women would face fewer work-based obstacles to establishing breastfeeding routines. Legislative interventions require support from policy makers and take time to pass and implement.

Although legislative interventions have broad application, they often target sites in addition to practices. So, for example, laws that prohibit hospitals and doctors from offering infant formula to mothers of newborns are forms of health intervention that are more focused than educating all mothers that they should breastfeed as soon as they can after giving birth or that they should reject infant formula at this time.

Social scientists interested in legislative interventions point out that they almost invariably involve struggles between competing interest groups, with significant resources at stake. For example, the legislative changes that altered the sales tactics of the Nestlé company in its worldwide distribution of infant formula in hospitals came about largely because of consumer pressure. A Nestlé product boycott spread throughout the world between 1977 and 1984; fighting it cost the company between $40 and $100 million (*Financial Times*, January 27, 1984:4; *Washington Post*, January 27, 1984:A1). In the end the company changed its infant formula marketing practices.

But legislation is far from a perfect form of intervention. Cigarettes and illicit drugs are widely available to minors in the United States despite being illegal. And although payments by cigarette companies following the tobacco settlement in the United States were supposed to be used by states to fund smoking interventions, they have instead been reappropriated by state governments to support general expenses ranging from health care to road building to education.

D. *Environmental Interventions*

Environmental interventions change physical space, or the use of physical space, so as to link a desired outcome inextricably with some practice. For example, if the objective is to reduce traffic fatalities, environmental interventions can modify how cars behave in accidents (how they brake, whether they have air bags, what force it takes to collapse a steering column). They also can influence how likely it is that roads themselves expose people to mortal hazards from bridge abutments, confusing lane mergers, or oncoming traffic. Because environmental interventions take choice out of the picture, when well-designed they can be extraordinarily effective. Iodizing salt and adding Vitamin D to milk are good examples of such environmental interventions. On a larger scale, chlorinating and fluoridating water at a central source is more effective than trying to educate people to add it at their homes, assuming the integrity of the delivery system.

The involuntary and public character of environmental interventions makes them especially contentious, even as it makes them particularly effective. In sites where health is thought to be an individual attribute, subject to individual rights, state manipulation of public behavior is viewed with deep suspicion. Thus the history of public health interventions in the United States is filled with examples of citizens asserting that government regulations about smoking, fluoride, vaccinations, or use of seatbelts impede their freedom and right to choose. This discomfort with state-sponsored limits to behavior may be one reason why such interventions are not more popular in epidemiologic thinking in the United States. On the other hand, relative comfort with a strong state role in public health make disease surveillance and environmental interventions more acceptable in countries like Denmark, Germany, and Japan. Debates about whether government has a legitimate right to limit individual freedom are a cultural component of decision-making about environmental interventions.

But other factors also restrict the use of environmental interventions. As noted earlier, the category *place* is still poorly conceptualized and measured in epidemiology. This hinders public health thinking about place-based interventions, where designers might think about how physical context gives behavioral cues and channels human social relationships in certain directions. Here one might envision which neighborhood layouts are likeliest to lead to social network formation among residents or how to design nursing homes that will maximize the comfort of Alzheimer's patients.

Political forces also impede development of some types of environmental interventions. Despite the emerging evidence about the broad and strong influence of poverty and inequality on health, for example, interventions that would change resource distribution, wealth accumulation, or zoning practices are branded as "social engineering" or "class warfare" rather than as sound public health policy. These types of interventions constrain the wealthy and powerful in ways that educational interventions do not, and they are therefore more threatening.

E.   Other Intervention Categories

From an anthropological perspective, the restricted use of environmental interventions is just one manifestation of a larger problem: that of categorization. Employing a framework in which interventions are said to "work" at four levels leads to its own limited set of recommendations. And thinking of interventions only in terms of these four levels limits our ability to pay attention to power (for example) as a central organizing principle of health intervention design. That is, structural interventions often work because they challenge and reframe both conventional behavior and conventional wisdom about where change takes place. Interventions work to the extent that they create new resources as well as new expectations, but new resources can be more difficult to find when one's attention is focused on just one type of managerial or knowledge-based solution.

The efficacy of interventions is greater when they take place at multiple levels to reinforce behavior change. The case of creative condom promotion is a brilliant example of mixing intervention types to promote cultural change. In Thailand, Mechai Viravaidya was the source of many creative and effective interventions to deal with birth control and AIDS prevention. When HIV/AIDS first came to Thailand, Mechai was already an important figure in family planning, and he used that knowledge and status to design AIDS interventions. Mechai used humor to approach sensitive areas of health behavior such as sex. For example, for many years his organization ran a restaurant called "Cabbages and Condoms" that had a bowl of free condoms at the cash register, where one might customarily expect to find a plate of mints. To reduce the mystique and illicit overtones of condoms, he sponsored condom-inflating contests in rural villages, in which prestigious elderly men competed. To help prospective clients of sex workers get exposed to AIDS prevention messages, his organization distributed condom education tapes to taxi drivers and asked them to play them on their car stereos whenever clients requested rides to houses of prostitution. A program called "Cops and Rubbers" gave condoms to policemen to distribute on New Year's Eve. Mechai and his colleagues were so successful in promoting condom use in Thailand that condoms are now called "mechais." The rate of AIDS increase has slowed in Thailand but not in neighboring countries, where AIDS control policies are more conservative and less creative.

Deciding which to choose among the four categories of educational, managerial, legislative, and environmental interventions implies making judgments about what can be changed and what cannot, who has power and who does not. The behavioral theories behind most interventions assume that individuals are the controlling force and agent of change. Create a disposition to change in an individual, the theory goes, and you can then offer specific instructions to that individual for how that change can be accomplished. But Ronald Frankenberg (1993) has suggested that when risk is seen as individual, it becomes something that people other than doctors (particularly patients) must do something about. He has pointed out that other aspects of risk get distributed across the professions involved in disease prevention and then become their responsibilities: clinical aspects of risk are perceived to be the domain of doctors and nurses, social aspects of risk are the domain of policy makers, and nonmodifiable aspects of risk like age or history are the domain of health educators who use them to mark their targets (Frankenberg 1993:230). This limits creative work on new intervention strategies and overemphasizes the power of individuals to create long-lasting change by themselves.

Medical anthropologists have undertaken educational, managerial, legislative, and environmental interventions, but they also have asked whether other categories of intervention might be equally compelling. For example, Corbett (2001) uses a social ecological framework to describe tobacco interventions at individual, group, organization, community, and population levels. And when Parker et al. (2000) describe international research on HIV prevention, they group structural and environmental factors together, paying particular attention to categories of economic underdevelopment and poverty, mobility, seasonal work, social disruption from war and political instability, gender inequality, and the effects of governmental and intergovernmental policies. Structural interventions require paying just as much attention to local context as do managerial or educational interventions, and one important contextual question in the international domain is whether an intervention can be equally successful in areas with many resources versus those with few to none.

The anthropologist Mary Douglas has asked why more attention has not been paid to the role institutions play in focusing human concern on low-probability events with dramatic consequences, rather than high-probability events with more mundane consequences (Douglas 1992:55–60). For example, how are people led to pay so much attention to deaths from airplane crashes and so little to the much more common problem of deaths from auto accidents? Why are a few deaths from Ebola virus so much more frightening than millions of deaths from malnutrition? This theme will be explored more fully in the next chapter.

II.   The Community in Public Health Interventions

*A.   The Difference between Intervening with Individuals
and Populations*

One of the most important ideas in the development of community interventions is that sustained attention must be devoted to the determinants
of disease incidence in populations. This idea has best been championed
by the British epidemiologist Geoffrey Rose. In 1985 Rose explored the
difference between thinking about the causes and prevention of disease
in specific individuals as compared with the causes and prevention of disease in populations. Rose pointed out that much of epidemiology consists
of case-control and cohort studies that measure differences between sick
and healthy individuals. But these studies take it for granted that exposure is heterogeneous in a population – if all individuals smoked, then
lung cancer could not be attributed to smoking. Rose then challenged his
readers to consider how to handle instances where an entire population is
exposed to some disease determinant. He pointed out that only comparisons across populations, or changes within populations over time, can
reveal this type of influence, not simply comparisons of sick to healthy
individuals within a population.

How is this relevant to intervention design? Rose identified two design approaches: the "high-risk" strategy and the "population" strategy.
The high-risk strategy is based on identifying individuals who, based on
screening for symptoms or behaviors, are likely to develop some disease
in the future. Specific strategies are then created for these individuals,
who are motivated to follow them because they know that otherwise they
are at particularly high risk to develop a disease. Smoking cessation programs for smokers who have trouble breathing and dietary interventions
for people who are obese and feel faint both follow this process of identifying individuals at risk and working with them to reduce their risks.

The population strategy works differently. As Rose put it, "This is the
attempt to control the determinants of incidence, to lower the mean level
of risk factors, to shift the whole distribution of exposure in a favourable
direction" (Rose 1985:37). Rather than identifying and intervening on
specific individuals at high risk of developing disease, the population approach tries to reduce risk for all by changing the environment or changing
general norms of behavior. This is effective because exposure is reduced
for a very large number of people. Reducing risk slightly for all can prevent
more cases than reducing risk significantly among a few. And reducing
risk for all also makes future cases less probable, something the individual
approach does not address.

The emphasis on population interventions has some subtle but profound implications for standard anthropological approaches to intervention design. With the exception of those who employ a political-economic perspective, medical anthropologists have tended to work on interventions among marginalized and minority individuals, those belonging to groups identified as having specific increased risk of disease because of their social position. But Rose urged a shift in this emphasis toward smaller risk reduction strategies in the population at large. He admitted that both strategies would be needed for the foreseeable future, but he saw the biggest public health payoffs coming from the population approach.

One anthropological caveat to Rose is to point out that the notion of "population" among humans is a problematic concept in its own right and should not be taken for granted. We saw the arbitrariness of many place- and person-based boundaries described in Chapter 4 and the influence of political boundaries on mean cholera case fatality rates in Chapter 5. It is not at all straightforward to decide what the relevant boundaries of human populations should be, especially if the goal is to compare a variety of exposures among them. Population-based interventions that take the boundaries of towns or provinces for granted may be challenged by the diverse meanings and contexts of health behaviors within those boundaries.

B.   How Community Changes Influence Individual Changes

When epidemiologists and other public health specialists design interventions for entire communities, they have opportunities to learn more about how community processes both inhibit and promote individual behavior change: "More detailed analyses of community change processes are needed because we understand very little about them, but they appear to have important effects on individual behavior" (Fortmann et al. 1995:582). Such statements are a call for the contextual and processual data that anthropology can produce, as shown in Benjamin Paul's pioneering volume on medical anthropology, *Health, Culture, and Community: Case Studies of Public Reactions to Health Programs*, published in 1955. Many of the chapters in this book have documented the reactions of groups around the world to health interventions ranging from mental health education to cholera vaccines to cooperative health associations. Analyses of legislation, political movements, media themes, and the ways in which popular concerns are manifested in protests, jokes, and songs are just a few of the ways by which anthropologists and other social scientists assess the relationships between mass culture and individual action. Detailed observational studies of human behavior over time complement the broad understandings of such behavior given by surveys or analyses of textual content. In fact some public health researchers have written that interventions designed to produce broad social and political changes must include qualitative evaluation components to assess their impact completely (McKinlay 1993, Smedley and Syme 2000:27). Multidisciplinary research allows an intervention's effects to be traced through the many different connections between community and individual.

Because of their complexity and expense, only a few broad community-based intervention studies exist, but they have provided many important conclusions about the feasibility and complexity of undertaking community-wide interventions. Successful cardiovascular disease prevention programs in Finland in the 1970s and 1980s were based on a community intervention project in the province of North Karelia, where the community itself first requested the intervention (Puska et al. 1998). The intervention aimed to lower blood pressure, smoking, and cholesterol levels and to improve diets in the population at large. It involved not just the health system, but also industry, schools, and voluntary organizations. It succeeded in lowering cardiovascular disease rates in the first decade of the study and cancer rates in the second, showing the gains attainable through population-based interventions.

The success of the North Karelia Project prompted other community-based interventions. The best-known in the United States are probably the Three Communities Study (Farquhar et al. 1977) and the Stanford Five-City Project (Fortmann and Varady 2000), both of which took place in California in the 1970s and 1980s. Like Karelia, these projects were explicitly designed to influence a broad population rather than specific audiences such as patients in hospitals, smokers, or people with heart disease. But these projects paid more explicit attention to communication theories. To amplify the effects of messages, they tried to stimulate interpersonal discussion within communities and thereby increase their diffusion. Radio, television, print media, and other printed materials were used to distribute information, but community groups and various coalitions also were mobilized in support of the project goals. Considerable efforts were expended to match messages and media types to different audiences.

Community interventions to change health risk factors have left researchers with many questions about complex communities:

Perhaps the most important lesson we have learned about communities is that there is much we do not know. Much public health intervention research has focused on the individual as the target of the change and of the intervention. Yet a consideration of communities as the units of intervention demands an understanding of the many elements within a community that influence individuals and their health behaviors. An integration of the multiple components of a community, its families, networks, institutions, and policies, allows researchers not only to understand each component more completely but also to determine the role of each component in influencing individual health behavior. (Fortmann et al. 1995:583)

The Five-City Project group acknowledged the importance of working with both formal and informal networks of power, understanding cultural differences within communities, and understanding how and why chronic diseases come to be concentrated among the poor. Interventions at community scale require adjusting research objectives to local goals and constraints: the Five-City researchers mentioned the need to work within communities; the importance of researchers giving up some power over content, type, and scope of interventions; and the significance of mobilizing residents to change their own rules and regulations (Fortmann et al. 1995:583). The list of research topics they identified as essential to further progress in community intervention design is basically a set of social science research issues:

- what knowledge, attitudes, behaviors, and communication patterns exist among population subgroups;
- how organizations, in addition to individuals, respond to interventions;
- how media organizations convey health information; and
- how, and under what pressures, local health-related policy initiatives develop.

In essence, when the entire community is the site of a health intervention, researchers must learn not only what individuals can do, but also what existing groups and organizations can do, and what they may not be willing to allow. Researchers involved in community interventions need to understand how information and behavioral expectations travel across social networks, and how political forces and legal frameworks support or impede change.

Given the specificity of the intervention and the potential breadth of the response, anthropological involvement in community intervention can serve not only the health-related objectives of the intervention but also the knowledge-based objectives of social scientists studying community development. For example, the work of two community health organizations in Hartford, Connecticut (the Hispanic Health Council and the Institute of Community Research), has been interdisciplinary but also heavily anthropological. Researchers at these groups were critical participants in creating a community-directed syringe exchange program to reduce HIV transmission (Singer 2001, 2003) and in assessing HIV risk among older urban adults (Radda et al. 2003). They have asked how structural factors (such as stratification, service availability, and quality) influence the spread of AIDS, and how social marginalization of various types (racial hatred, class discrimination, sexism, even daily indignities) manifests itself in a variety of forms of social misery (Singer 2001). Singer suggests that research on substances like alcohol, tobacco, and drugs is a fruitful opportunity for collaboration within traditional anthropological subfields of cultural, physical, and linguistic anthropology, as well as archaeology, and that it takes anthropology "into the bright light of direct encounter with issues of pressing public concern" (2001:210–211). Surely intentional public health interventions also can serve to diagnose societies, because, like disease outbreaks, they create different kinds of reactions from the competing factions and interest groups that live together in communities.

III.   Anthropological Participation in Population Interventions

As epidemiologists and public health researchers get more involved in community interventions, they face challenges extending beyond their customary disciplinary boundaries. Epidemiologists have acknowledged their need to expand their expertise: for example, the theme for the 1998 annual meeting of the American College of Epidemiology was "Epidemiology and Community Interventions in Diverse Populations." Yet anthropologists, who ostensibly understand a great deal about communities and diversity, have rarely had central roles in designing large-scale community health interventions.

Community interventions provide at least two different opportunities for anthropologists: roles as brokers (mediators between cultures) and as designers. Anthropological knowledge of how groups form and manipulate ethnic and other identities allows them to become brokers between intervention designers and local communities. They have played this role for at least four decades, since the Johns Hopkins medical geography projects described in Chapter 2 and some of the studies published in Paul's (1955) book. But the culture broker role is increasingly problematic for outsiders because of the concerns about control and representativeness faced by any person claiming to be able to mediate between two different social groups. The culture broker role also takes as given that "culture" is the heart of the problem, when it may instead be place-based risks such as environmental contamination or policy environments (e.g., bank lending policies or welfare policies on daycare coverage) that place some groups at systematic disadvantage.

The designer role is likelier to offer greater impact for anthropologists in intervention projects. U.S. anthropologists have, in fact, developed many "culturally appropriate" intervention models at the scale of an urban neighborhood or rural village (Nastasi and Berg 1999). But with few exceptions, anthropologists have not participated as actively or often in the design and evaluation of interventions at larger scale. Many of those who have participated in population-level responses to public health challenges have been particularly interested in the political and economic determinants of health (e.g., Hall et al. 1999 on smoking policies among Northwest Indian tribes, Nichter et al. 1997 and Ernster et al. 2000 on women and smoking, Singer 2001 on needle exchange programs, and Stebbins 1997 on smoking control legislation in West Virginia). This is because population-level interventions require theoretical orientations that take account of large-scale structural change. Medical anthropologists with a political-economic orientation are better prepared to see opportunities and develop strategies to create such change.

Many anthropologists have strong views about the perils of planned change by supra-local institutions of government, religion, and commerce. Their experiences tend to make them suspicious of initiatives planned from above without extensive participation by local communities. But to date most health interventions *do* arrive from above: they are produced by experts with extensive data about the risks particular practices pose to health. They are imposed by bureaucrats and scientists who assume that health is everyone's first priority, and that all people define health in basically the same way.

Much as epidemiologists have learned that community interventions must adapt to local conditions, so anthropologists have argued that planned change in communities must begin with extensive community consultations, emerge from local definitions of need, and be continuously subject to local review and adjustment over time (e.g., Nastasi and Berg 1999). These requirements conflict with those community health interventions that specify in advance the desired health-related goals, the behaviors needing change, and the messages required to prompt such changes. As more health-related interventions take place at larger scale, there will be more opportunities for anthropologists to become involved in the types of consultative processes they champion. The next sections describe studies by anthropologists in Brazil and Bangladesh that adapted professional health-related objectives to existing contexts and practices in the general population.

A.   Designing a Provider Intervention in Brazil

The Northeast is one of the poorest areas in Brazil; diarrheal disease there is the most important cause of death among children under five years of age. Oral rehydration solution (ORS) is the most effective treatment for dehydration caused by diarrhea; it can be prepared by mixing water with glucose, sodium chloride, sodium bicarbonate, and potassium chloride. Foil-wrapped packets are the form of ORS preferred by the World Health Organization and by almost all physicians: these are easily dispensed and stored, and they provide and regulate the ratio of most of the key ingredients in the solution. On the other hand packets are not always available, and they keep control of therapy in professional hands rather than mothers'. A solution of salt, sugar, and water easily mixed in the home is less expensive but quite close to the packet form of ORS, and mothers simply can be urged to give extra liquids to sick children.

Anthropologists in Brazil believed that ORS should be introduced as a simple household procedure rather than as a hospital-based, medically controlled intervention (Nations et al. 1988). They considered how to introduce oral rehydration therapy in a simpler and more culturally sensitive fashion than the medicalized packets. The Northeast has one doctor for every 2000 patients, but it has one traditional healer for every 150 patients. So the anthropologists trained traditional healers to add salt and sugar in specified ratios to the medicinal teas they already offered their patients with diarrhea. The herbs included in the teas (often chamomile and peppermint) did not hinder the absorption of the liquid. With just slight modifications to their customary practices, the healers adapted familiar treatments to meet international standards.

B.   Designing a Household Intervention in Bangladesh

In the 1980s, fieldworkers at the International Centre for Diarrheal Disease Research in Bangladesh were searching for ways to standardize the proportions of sugar, salt, and water used by village women to prepare sugar-salt solution. They learned that a large number of container sizes existed within villages, and it was difficult to find a standard-size container in which to measure water. They adapted to local constraints by asking mothers to bring their metal water vessels to a group meeting. Then they filled a standard liter bottle of water and transferred its contents, in turn, into each container brought by the women. Marking the water line inside the container with a nail created a standard measure within existing containers, a simple solution to a vexing problem.

C.   Interventions and Authority

There are many ways to reach individuals, and some of them take advantage of the power of social influence. When risk becomes familial or regional, then it becomes something for families and entire populations to confront. An intervention to increase water hygiene, for example, can begin with general messages to drink boiled water, and specific messages about how long water must be boiled before it can be considered fit for drinking. These messages are targeted primarily at household caretakers, almost invariably women. Other intervention campaigns are directed to whole villages, neighborhoods, towns, or cities. "This is what it means to live here as a member of this community," such messages say, "This is how we live, and if you live here you should try to act this way, too." Interventions can take the form of political campaigns urging supporters to demand their rights to clean water, adequate health services, or sufficient food.

Health campaigns often rely on the authority of professionals to urge the populace to change its use of medications. Other public health campaigns urge the populace to stop smoking, drink responsibly, use condoms, wear seatbelts, brush teeth, or thoroughly cook meat. Intervention designers rely on various sources of authority when they call for these practices. They employ the authority of science – that scientific studies "show" that continuing practice X increases risk of outcome Y. They employ the authority of government, urging citizens to comply because policy X is more effective and less costly than policy Y. And they employ the authority of medicine, that doctors say practice Z is healthier.

The next section looks at one source of authority for the health practices recommended by intervention designers: it describes sociocultural influences on the "gold standard" research design, the randomized controlled trial.

IV.   The Tools of Intervention Research: An Anthropological Analysis of Randomized Controlled Trials

A.   How Patient and Physician Expectations Influence the Conduct of Randomized Controlled Trials

Epidemiology today is a primary source of the research designs relied on to produce authoritative proof of the efficacy of some new intervention. Randomized controlled trials (RCTs) are considered the most convincing form of epidemiologic data about treatment efficacy. But RCTs are a technology rather than a source of truth. This section argues that better understanding of the sociocultural components of RCTs will yield more qualified acceptance of their power and better understanding of their limits.

In their simplest form, RCTs (called "clinical trials" when specifically testing clinical interventions) start with a group of similar people with a treatable health condition. These people are randomly allocated either to receive a treatment (the experimental group) or no treatment (the control group), and then they are followed over time while their response to treatment is measured. Randomization is undertaken not to make both groups equal but rather to evenly distribute both known and unknown factors that might influence response to treatment. Some RCTs also include a group of people receiving a placebo, a substance similar to the treatment substance in all ways except that it is designed to have no treatment efficacy. RCTs use placebos to try to measure what part of a treatment's effects might be attributable solely to a patient's expectations that the treatment will be effective (see Moerman 2002).

RCTs are filled with sociocultural components. To begin with, they are feasible only under certain social conditions. Undertaking a randomized controlled trial is justified when there is a social and professional consensus that an unanswered research question is important and that not enough is known to warrant giving or withholding a treatment from all patients. By the time that happens, the issue may have been well vetted in the media, and people may have formed opinions about it. (This is the case, e.g., with large-scale interventions to reduce smoking or heart disease.) Individuals and entire communities may therefore debate and change their practices even while a trial is getting underway. This "awareness effect" can change the behavior of both experimental and control groups at the same time, reducing the likelihood that an intervention will produce notable improvement in experimental groups compared with controls. There is an obvious paradox inherent in the fact that the same conditions that make a controlled trial possible also can create difficulties in analyzing whether it has been successful.

Because clinical trials compare new treatments with existing treatments, or with none at all, the experimental treatment must offer some possibility of improvement over the existing accepted treatments or standards. Otherwise it would be ethically impossible to justify randomly allocating the treatment to part of a population. When a therapy is especially promising and an illness particularly dangerous, trials must be designed so that they can be stopped as soon as a new treatment appears to be effective. That is, when scientific consensus emerges *during* a clinical trial that the experimental treatment is effective, the trial must be altered so that the treatment also can be provided to the control group.

Surveillance committees have been created for this purpose; they follow treatment results and make decisions about whether an early halt to a study might be appropriate. The need to stop an RCT because of proof of efficacy demonstrates that health improvement is valued over research outcomes. The belief that people should not serve as guinea pigs for science partly springs from recent events in which they did (for example, the Tuskegee syphilis study that involved withholding treatment over decades to infected but uninformed African American men, as well as the Nazi medical experiments performed on concentration camp prisoners).

If, as part of their rationale, controlled trials require scientific uncertainty about proper treatment, they also depend on public consensus that participation in a trial brings potential benefits and justifiable risks to the participant. The pharmaceutical industry is a major source of funding for RCTs, and pharmaceutical companies are increasingly having for-profit research firms run these trials rather than teaching hospitals and medical schools. Patient enrollment practices have been questioned as corporate profits become more important than the search for knowledge. Pharmaceutical research also is complex these days because advocacy groups apply pressure on pharmaceutical companies and the federal government to develop new treatments. These groups try to track the availability of new treatments that might be useful for their members, and many even maintain databases showing what types of patients are still needed to fulfill enrollment requirements for ongoing clinical trials. One quite new force in the clinical trial process is the presence of patient advocacy groups such as ACT UP for AIDS patients (Löwy 2000), or Little People of America or the National Marfan Association in new genetic therapy research (Rapp et al. 2001). When antiretroviral medications were first being tested on HIV patients, joining a clinical trial advertised by a patient advocacy group was the best way to get treatment. In this case, however, patients were really only interested in joining the group likely to receive treatment, which conflicts with the study's randomization component.

One way researchers deal with this pressure is to create designs where patients "cross over" from one study arm to the other after a predetermined period. People first assigned to receive active medications might later be switched to placebos instead, whereas those in the placebo arm would later get active treatment. In this variant of the "research as social exchange model" the researchers are creating designs to respond to patients' desire for treatments. Patients want some treatment rather than no treatment, even when the treatment has not been proven effective and may turn out to be harmful.

A similar dynamic can be seen when research staff fail to describe study options equally to potential enrollees. This is particularly important when a randomized controlled trial includes an intensive monitoring arm in addition to treatment arms because many sick people are unlikely to accept equal chances that they will receive an intervention or nothing at all. How potential research subjects think about consenting or refusing to participate in an RCT is still poorly understood. One in-depth qualitative study based on interviews with parents of critically ill newborns who were asked to participate in a clinical trial showed that they often did not understand the randomization process or its rationale (Snowdon et al. 1997). Furthermore, research staff sometimes inadvertently allowed parents to assume they were promoting a new treatment over conventional treatment. An innovative design in England explored and resolved this dilemma by embedding a trial within a qualitative research project. In-depth interviews explored how study recruiters interpreted study information, and audiotape recordings of actual recruitment sessions explored how recruiters presented study information. The researchers found that early in the study the recruiters presented the active treatment options first, describing them as aggressive and curative, whereas they presented the monitoring last and described it as "watchful waiting" (Donovan et al. 2002:768). As the analysis progressed, recommendations for how to change presentation strategies were circulated to all the study centers. Among the many changes suggested was a substitution of the phrase "active monitoring" for the prior "watchful waiting." Over time patients' willingness to be randomized to any study arm increased from 40% of those approached to 70%. The study methods also allowed the researchers to explore other ways in which the confidence of recruiters influenced patient decisions.

B.   *Why RCT Designs Limit Intervention Possibilities*

RCTs play a large role in "evidence-based medicine," a trend linking contemporary research and clinical practice in which significant treatments are assessed using clinical trials and then compared according to their cost and efficacy. The power of RCT designs is both statistical and social. Analyses of aggregate datasets describing multiple groups of people from different study populations (so-called meta-analyses) often limit their data sources to clinical trials so that only the most robust findings are analyzed. This restricts the theoretical models that can be employed and the types of data that become admissible as evidence.

RCTs are a new type of technology in epidemiology, popular especially in the past three decades. Those who do cultural studies of science have pointed out that although new technology often allows new things to be seen, it also facilitates an interpretation that what one has newly seen is something that is "natural" rather than something translated through the technology. The difficulty of using RCTs to study the health impact of social networks, neighborhoods, and inequality makes these influences seem unproven, and therefore less "scientific." But in fact it is the mismatch between the theme and the research design that makes the data difficult to obtain, not some underlying weakness in the theme.

The historical exclusion of women from many clinical trials of cardiovascular disease until the 1980s is another example of how technology makes results seem "natural." Because the female risk was perceived to be low, it was measured infrequently and allowed to become largely invisible. The U.S. National Institutes of Health are now trying to eliminate such imbalances, making executive rulings (a form of administrative intervention) that force researchers to include all potential groups at risk or to justify any exclusions. We are likely to see more "health problems" and new risks among women, minorities, and children in the future, not because there are new epidemics and risks but because these groups were neglected in past research.

All intervention trials that involve randomized controlled designs face a common challenge. To distribute baseline differences evenly among individuals or communities, they must randomly assign individuals or communities to either intervention or control groups. But if statistical analyses are to be valid, the unit of randomization must be the same as the unit of analysis. When individuals are randomized to an intervention, results should be based on statistics about individuals, as in the proportion of individuals responding to experimental treatment X compared with those responding to placebo Y. And when groups or communities or cities are randomized to interventions, then groups or communities or cities should be the unit of analysis. This creates two problems. First, randomization of a limited number of communities to intervention and control groups does not guarantee equal distribution of baseline characteristics among individuals in those communities. Second, the health outcomes of individuals in a community receiving an intervention should not be seen as independent of one another, although the statistical tests used to compare rates among individuals commonly assume such independence (Kirkwood et al. 1997).

If whole communities are chosen as units of intervention and researchers are interested in the average level of some outcome variable like cardiovascular disease rates, analyses should first aggregate those rates by community. Then the distribution of those rates can be compared across intervention and control communities. This design requirement has dramatic implications for study complexity and cost, since randomizing 10 or 16 or 30 communities and managing separate interventions in half of them is far more complex than assuming one can count all individuals in one community as "experimental" subjects and all the individuals in the other as "control" subjects. If a study includes one intervention community and one control community, it really has just two units of study, not the total number of individuals in those two units.

Researchers have developed ways to deal with the statistical and design issues confronting community-based interventions. One can take multiple measures of change in each community over time, for example, or match each intervention community with a control community, or compare those within each community who adopt the intervention with those who do not (for additional options, see Kirkwood et al. 1997). But these complexities themselves are another reason why controlled trials of community interventions are uncommon.

RCTs often are not useful for assessing social and economic influences on health. In the 1970s and 1980s there were large RCTs in the United States of income maintenance, housing allowances, and worker training programs (Oakely 1998). But these were generally outside the health field, tested alternative program designs, and analyzed data at the level of the individual rather than the community. The cost and complexity of controlled trials further limit the types of research questions they are generally employed to answer. Complex social forces like social networks, neighborhood effects, or social inequality cannot be randomly assigned to individuals, and they cannot be withheld.

On the other hand, medication effects, surgical outcomes, and even some types of behavioral interventions can readily be evaluated using RCT designs. The Centers for Disease Control and Prevention has recently begun to evaluate preventive interventions (*Guide to Community Preventive Services*), giving high priority to data from randomized trials just like evidence-based medicine. But some experts predict that as a result the *Guide* will contain fewer data on true community interventions and more on interventions directed at individuals or small groups (Green and Kreuter 2000).

One form of RCT increasingly used in studies of global health is the multicenter RCT. Multicenter RCTs involve gathering large numbers of patients from different research centers, sometimes even across multiple countries, applying the same intervention in each site, and then evaluating the intervention's effect based on the pooled populations of all experimental subjects and all controls across all the sites at once. They decrease the time required to carry out the trial and increase the generalizability and power of the results. Multicenter RCT designs also impose limitations on researchers. For example, patients at a site actually can come from a broad range of social and cultural backgrounds. But patient variety attributable to differences across contributing centers is seen more as a hindrance than a benefit because the more varied the patients are, the harder it is to generalize across them. So efforts are made to keep study protocols and intervention processes as simple and standardized as possible. This limits the types of interventions that are capable of being assessed in this format, and it limits local researchers' abilities to adapt global interventions to their local contexts. Only certain types of interventions can pass through this new and popular form of epidemiologic assessment. The design drives the types of questions that can be asked, rather than the other way around.

Because the RCT is such an important and respected technology, it has the power to dictate the types of interventions that are recommended (specifically because they have been proven in controlled trials) or not (e.g., those that cannot be easily assessed through controlled trials). The RCT is indeed a powerful tool, but this section has argued that overreliance on it as the most authoritative source of evidence can have the effect of limiting the imagination and impeding public health progress.

V.   Conclusion

Opportunities for partnership among social scientists and epidemiologists are pervasive when public health interventions move to address population-level contexts and concerns. Today's interventions are increasingly designed to be collaborative: research topics address issues of mutual concern, potential participants are involved in the study design, and those who design intervention strategies are less presumptuous about anticipating the "correct" direction of behavioral change that ought to result. These are positive trends from an anthropological point of view, for anthropologists have long suggested that local populations and affected individuals must be involved in intervention projects. It is therefore gratifying to see that many community-based health interventions take place today only after local professionals and residents have had a chance to comment on and revise procedures.

On the other hand, anthropologists also would predict that any recommendation to change behavior would encounter opposition from those stakeholders who benefit from its presence. Even when produced collaboratively by local professionals and residents, those television campaigns to reduce smoking, drinking, and obesity that I see on television at 3 A.M. in foreign cities are more than offset by the evening advertisements for cigarettes, alcohol, and fast food stores.

This chapter continues the theme – woven throughout this book – that epidemiological assumptions, techniques, and conclusions reflect sociocultural influences. Health intervention projects may be the most significant and most problematic use of contemporary epidemiology. As intervention designs focus more on environmental interventions and legislation, their impact becomes at once broader and larger. Recommended revisions of legislation and modifications of environment are more widespread and far-reaching, and therefore more controversial or confusing. The public can interpret controversial recommendations as uncertainty rather than advancement, reducing or complicating the efficacy of some intervention initiatives. This dilemma is explored in the next chapter.

FOR FURTHER READING

Hahn R., ed. 1999. *Anthropology in Public Health*. Oxford: Oxford University Press.

Paul B. D., ed. 1955. *Health, Culture, and Community: Case Studies of Public Reactions to Health Programs*. New York: Russell Sage Foundation.

Rose G. 1992. *The Strategy of Preventive Medicine*. Oxford: Oxford University Press.

Smedley B. D. and S. L. Syme, eds. 2000. *Promoting Health: Intervention Strategies from Social and Behavioral Research. Institute of Medicine*. Washington, DC: National Academy Press.

Sobo E. J. 1995. *Choosing Unsafe Sex: AIDS-risk Denial among Disadvantaged Women*. Philadelphia: University of Pennsylvania Press.

7   Perceiving and Representing Risk

Epidemiologists came under increasingly critical public scrutiny in the 1990s. In 1993 the *Lancet* published an editorial with the provocative heading "Do epidemiologists cause epidemics?" It inquired whether epidemiologists were making too many errors in their calculations of disease burden and causation, and whether the public was placing excessive confidence in – and deriving excessive anxiety from – epidemiological results. A 1995 news report in the journal *Science*, titled "Epidemiology faces its limits," began with this devastating sentence: "The news about health risks comes thick and fast these days, and it seems almost constitutionally contradictory" (Taubes 1995:164). As the cartoon in Figure 7.1 makes clear, epidemiology has increasing presence in the mass media, but its recommendations for how to maintain health and avoid disease seem arbitrary and subject to rapid change. Yet people seek more information about risk even if they do not quite know what it is.

Epidemiology has, until recently, been an accepted source of evidence in many countries about how to identify and reduce disease risk. But that disciplinary authority is increasingly contested by representatives of private industry, government, and the public, who struggle to establish their own definitions of risk and rational solutions to the problem of risk. Because their messages are no longer broadcast only within the profession, epidemiologists' growing engagement in public affairs raises the stakes for the discipline. This public engagement is beginning to cause a struggle over how epidemiologists should present their claims and how much control they can or should exert over the dissemination of scientific findings.

I.   Popular and Professional Ideas about Risk

Anthropological research on classification and knowledge production can help shed light on this problem. In addition to their descriptions of disease burden, epidemiologists and other public health scientists produce public messages about one key topic: risk. Risk is the rhetorical vehicle

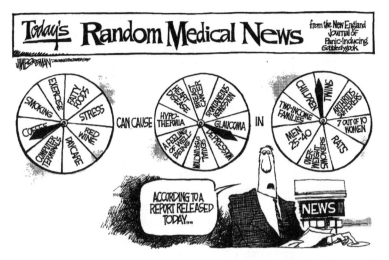

Figure 7.1. Medical news cartoon. Borgman, J. *The Cincinnati Inquirer*, 1997. Reprinted with special permission of King Features Syndicate.

health scientists use to project the past and the present into the future. As Paul Slovic, an American risk perception expert trained in psychology, points out,

Danger is real, but risk is socially constructed. Risk assessment is inherently subjective and represents a blending of science and judgment with important psychological, social, cultural, and political factors.... Whoever controls the definition of risk controls the rational solution to the problem at hand. If you define risk one way, then one option will rise to the top as the most cost-effective, or the safest, or the best. If you define it another way, perhaps incorporating qualitative characteristics and other contextual factors, you will likely get a different ordering of your action solutions. Defining risk is thus an exercise in power. (Slovic 1997:95)

Popular and professional ideas about risk often differ. Laypeople appear to think they can live lives free of risk, whereas scientists face pressures to phrase their results in terms of risk instead of rates or ratios. It has been suggested that there is an epidemic of "risk" itself in clinical journals, going beyond new terminology to reflect changing cultural ideas about what factors lie under human control (Skolbekken 1995). Because risk, menace, and safety are an inherent part of what health scientists communicate to the public, their communication of these concepts must be improved.

Risk is the concept used by health scientists to transform a series of individual disease states (e.g., smokers who get lung cancer and nonsmokers who get lung cancer) into a single group measure (e.g., relative risk of getting lung cancer for smokers compared with nonsmokers). Based on some particular study of living or deceased members of some population, epidemiologists produce estimates of the likelihood of future disease or dysfunction. Yet risk is a particularly problematic vehicle for conveying scientific data because it has clear but divergent meanings to scientists and the general public. Risk for scientists is an estimate of probability or likelihood of occurrence based on comparisons. Risk for the general public is a synonym of menace and danger: one takes risks, one risks one's life.

The statistical probabilities used to express risk do not make a great deal of intuitive sense to most individuals. One may be told one has a 10-fold increased risk of developing lung cancer as a smoker compared with a nonsmoker, but in the end a smoker gets cancer or does not, and a nonsmoker gets cancer or does not. Probabilities are not easily perceived; the unroped climber poised on a small rock crystal high above the ground senses danger because his fingers are beginning to tremble, not because he has some inherent sense that his lifetime probability of having a serious accident is 0.01. And that climber knows full well that his lifetime probability of dying is 1 – if he is to meet death early, why not have the encounter on his own terms? In this case the certainty of eventual death must be weighed against the certainty of present pleasure and possibility of early death. And so he adjusts his grip and keeps climbing. Up.

In some ways people do not seem to do a very good job at estimating the health risk posed by their environment or their behavior. They are anxious about (unlikely) large disasters with catastrophic consequences and forget about (quite probable) exposure to more common but smaller-scale accidents or health problems. That is, they worry more about dying in an airplane crash than dying in their car on the way to the airport, and they think nuclear radiation causes more cancer than radon gas. They are more concerned about the risks of their children having peanut allergies than of being obese. The media make much of new diseases such as West Nile virus, Lyme Disease, or SARS but do not sensationalize the real mass murderers called heart disease and cancer.

But, as the next section shows, in other ways people do an excellent job of estimating their risk. Their estimates of risk are strongly influenced by their social characteristics as well as their knowledge of a behavior or the comparison they are asked to make between behaviors. What motivates people to change is not the abstract risk of contracting a disease but rather the real risk a disease would pose to their plans and dreams (White 1999).

As we have seen throughout this book, it is complex and difficult to translate information about the acquisition of disease within populations into information about the avoidance of disease for individuals.

In fact, some of the most interesting recent work on risk communication comes from the disciplines of psychology, engineering, and public policy, where researchers are devoted both to understanding and bridging differences between professional and public worldviews of what is dangerous and what can be changed. These works represent high levels of interdisciplinarity: a "Mental Models Approach" to risk communication developed by engineers and psychologists (Morgan et al. 2002) looks similar to some of the social science efforts described in this chapter. A book attempting to show objective comparisons among 50 different types of risks (related to home or work, the environment, or health and medicine) uses both epidemiological and toxicological data (Ropeik and Gray 2002). And a special issue of the *British Medical Journal* (see Edwards 2003) contains articles written by clinicians, risk communication experts, sociologists, policy analysts, and others describing a variety of ways physicians can communicate risk levels to their patients. In short, many disciplinary voices are now talking about how best to transmit data on risk to the general population.

Popular and Lay Epidemiology

Descriptions of how epidemiologists gather data about risk would usually begin with the epidemiologists' top-down perspective. But here I would like to take a bottom-up approach in keeping with the theory that people create risk, perceptions of risk, and professional rules to manage and control knowledge about risk. So I begin with "popular epidemiology" and "lay epidemiology," two concepts relevant for increasing the discipline's engagement with the populace. The following sections briefly describe what these mean, and then they discuss some ways that anthropological research, and hybrid work in cultural epidemiology, might usefully extend these notions beyond their original territory.

Popular epidemiology was defined in 1992 as "the process by which laypersons gather scientific data and other information, and also direct and marshal the knowledge and resources of experts in order to understand the epidemiology of disease" (Brown 1992:269). There are strong precursors to this definition, for example, books written for nonprofessionals about how to investigate environmental hazards (Brown et al. 1990; Legator et al. 1985; Legator and Strawn 1993). Popular epidemiology grows out of the public's growing involvement in environmental health concerns. Community residents begin to share information about local health problems, link exposure to local pollutants, organize formal investigations, and interact with supportive and opposing groups in government, academe, and industry (Brown 1992:269–70).

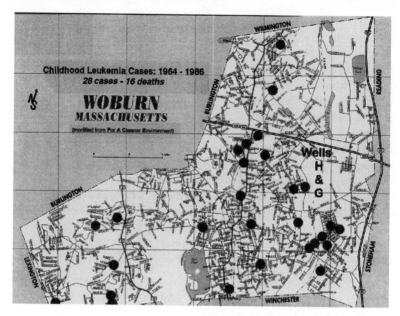

Figure 7.2. Distribution of childhood leukemia cases in Woburn, Massachusetts. Available online at: http://www.geology.ohio-state.edu/ courtroom/leuk41g.jpg. Woburn telephone directory map copyright by JFL Publishing.

Popular epidemiology sometimes starts with disease outbreaks represented on maps. Geographic descriptions of wind vectors and disease risk are familiar in studies of nuclear mishaps like the Chernobyl reactor meltdown or accidental chemical releases like Bhopal in India. But they also are important focal points for community self-study when neighborhood residents suspect the presence of cancer or other disease clusters.

Such a map played a central role in a famous lawsuit in Woburn, Massachusetts, fought over whether childhood leukemia cases were caused by toxic chemicals in local polluted wells. (See the book [Harr 1996] and the movie *A Civil Action*.) The case began when a mother began to map the presence of what she perceived to be surprisingly high numbers of children with leukemia in her neighborhood. That map (see Figure 7.2) played a key role in attracting the attention of scientists, lawyers, and public officials.

The map is particularly interesting because it prompts viewers to assume that these cases are clustered in time and space, and that the cluster has some connection to the two nearby wells. Note that the map contains no reference to the size of the underlying population or the length of exposure to the water, nor does it display the distribution of cases further away from the wells. Readers actually cannot use it to draw conclusions about whether these cases of childhood leukemia represent larger totals than what might be expected for a population of this size in this area. Yet it still prompts attention.

Maps draw attention in popular epidemiology because they represent data in familiar form. Unlike statistical data on risk and exposure, maps show readers where objects or people are located in relation to sites that they can see or readily imagine. Most people work with maps all their lives, so they know – or think they know – how to interpret their messages and meanings. A newspaper reporter made this point about local residents' construction of maps of breast cancer on Long Island, New York:

It started in a few small towns where the breast cancer rate seemed suspiciously high. Anxious residents would record new cases on homemade maps, noting their proximity to dry cleaners, factories, wells or anything else that might have made their neighbors sick. Now, lawmakers have set aside $1 million for a statewide cancer mapping project, the first of its kind in the nation. (Goodnough 1998:30)

This is another example where a homemade map creates initial attention and is followed by more rigorous and professional renditions of data.

Popular epidemiology promotes the public's use of scientific epidemiological methods. It justifies the public's role in studying health concerns before professionals give them (both the public *and* the concerns) credibility. But it does not promote using epidemiologic methods to study problems that fall outside professional definitions: "It is obviously necessary to evaluate the correctness of findings that result from popular epidemiology. Such knowledge is not 'folk' knowledge with an antiscientific basis. In most cases, popular epidemiology findings are the result of scientific studies involving trained professionals, even if they begin as 'lay mapping' of disease clusters without attention to base rates or controls" (Brown 1992:277–8). Popular epidemiology describes community mobilization to bring health issues to light, to involve epidemiologists in studies of these issues, and to collect relevant data with or without professional assistance.

Some epidemiologists *do* accept and promote using their methods to study lay health concerns. *Lay epidemiology* has been defined by an interdisciplinary British group as "a scheme in which individuals interpret health risks through the routine observation and discussion of cases of illness and death in personal networks and the public arena, as well as from formal and informal evidence arising from other sources, such as television and magazines" (Frankel et al. 1991:428). Lay epidemiology reflects people's deep awareness of some types of personal and short-term risks, for example, the increased likelihood that they will have an automobile accident if they drive while drunk. But Frankel and colleagues argue that people are less concerned by more distant and long-term risks, such as the increased risk of heart disease from excess fat consumption. They have more recently used the concept of lay epidemiology to argue that disadvantaged groups in industrialized countries are acting rationally by not stopping smoking because the act of smoking helps them cope with stress and they are necessarily more focused on survival in the short rather than the long term (Lawlor et al. 2003). Lay epidemiology thus emphasizes the validity of local knowledge about risk, knowledge that puts risk in context.

Some creative strategies have been developed that can be used to visualize lay epidemiology among rural and nonliterate populations. Robert Chambers' work with Participatory Rural Appraisal (PRA) is one of the best-known examples of using graphic forms of information collection and display in participatory evaluation in developing countries (Chambers 1997). PRA practitioners work with rural villagers to produce maps of crop use and soil quality, bar charts of seasonal differences in production and household income, and cluster diagrams of wealth ranking or medicinal uses of local plants. They do this through innovative strategies that rely on public production of data and use of available and familiar materials. For example, a PRA team might ask villagers to draw a map of their village in the dirt of the central square. They would ask passersby to check and improve it and might also ask them to use sticks or rocks to indicate household locations, land that is fertile and infertile, or places where children live who do not attend school. Over the course of a day an accurate map can be produced that can assist land use planning or school siting, or identify disabled children. Or they might ask locals to make a graph on the ground of a year's time, divided up into locally important units like months, climate changes, or growing seasons. They would then ask people to indicate during which seasons agricultural products were planted, harvested, or sold, when money was circulating or in short supply, when people tended to run out of food. Each of these diagrams (the first a map, the second a bar chart) subsequently could be transferred to paper for safekeeping.

Two important points can be made about this work: rural villagers are able to produce sophisticated graphic displays of their knowledge, and they can be treated as active participants in a research process rather than passive subjects of a research study. These mapping and graphing techniques require, or at least allow, a creative form of interaction between professional and villager or professor and student. When used to describe health-related data they form an interesting combination of popular and lay epidemiology: these methods can be used to represent a broad array of local health concerns, not only those of interest to visiting outsiders. But they also rely on local people and materials and knowledge to produce health-related data about their own specific place.

Anthropologists also have offered some good examples of the importance of lay epidemiology. Rayna Rapp's article about women's willingness to undergo amniocentesis uses the term "community epidemiology" for what has been called lay epidemiology here. (See also Rapp 1999.)

Many women without a high degree of scientific literacy have developed a practical sense of community epidemiology. Enfolding their own reproductive health into that of kin and friends, they say [about whether to undergo amniocentesis], "I don't smoke, I don't do drugs. My mother had my sister when she was forty, my sisters, they all had late babies, healthy babies. My friends, they're all fine. I'm healthy, I don't need this test." (Rapp 1998:154–155)

This kind of statement points to the (largely unnoticed) role that public interpretation of epidemiologic data already plays in guiding health behavior. The details of this process of interpretation may not quite conform to scientists' desires, but the process nonetheless resembles an active comparison between personal experience and external evidence.

The emergence of popular and lay epidemiology remind health scientists that they should pay more attention to types of knowledge and power that circulate outside of professional boundaries. But these two concepts represent different approaches to public engagement and public knowledge. To further emphasize this difference, we could call popular epidemiology "community-controlled epidemiology" and lay epidemiology "the epidemiology of local knowledge." Using the term "community-controlled epidemiology" emphasizes that expertise useful in standard epidemiological research projects also resides among those who are not professionally trained; using the term "epidemiology of local knowledge" emphasizes that epidemiological research methods also can be applied to nonbiomedical illness labels.

An Example of Community-Controlled epidemiology in Canada

Who has the right to measure and to construct "portraits" of sickness and health in communities? Epidemiology is a tool often used by the nation-state and dominant groups within nation-states to describe and define the health problems of the powerless. In Canada, an anthropologist and a group of aboriginal collaborators helped to shape a government epidemiology initiative to design a "National Longitudinal Aboriginal Health Survey" (O'Neil et al. 1998). They sought to make a survey that would improve on the more typical research approach to Native American communities, where outsiders describe these communities as sick, disorganized, and dependent.

As we saw in Chapter 6, it is dangerous to assume that a scientist works with one monolithic community rather than a community factionalized by competing voices and interests. For example, the Canadian group needed to account for the possibility that women would report and request services for health concerns that differed from those reported and requested by men. In similar fashion, aboriginal health workers who sought to reinforce local knowledge wanted to describe and measure local healing practices, but they also were concerned that questions about traditional healing might offend community members who followed evangelical Christian practices.

The design process began with a series of workshops in different Canadian cities to consult with aboriginal health technicians working with aboriginal organizations and communities (O'Neil et al. 1998). Most of the participants initially were critical of the notion that more research needed to be done on aboriginal communities, but they eventually voiced support for a health survey if aboriginal peoples maintained control of funds, question content, implementation, analysis, and dissemination. They wanted the survey to produce information that would be both trustworthy at the community level and credible to scientists and government officials.

To respond to these concerns, a set of regional surveys and regional steering committees was created. A core set of questions was developed for use in all regions, but opportunities were created for each region to add its own questions. The regional steering committees then contracted with local consultants and universities to undertake the survey work (First Nations and Inuit Regional Health Survey National Steering Committee 1999). In the province of Manitoba, for example, eight aboriginal university students were hired to interview key stakeholders about health issues and concerns in all 61 First Nations in the province (O'Neil et al. 1998). They were trained both by university researchers and by Tribal Councils.

In Manitoba, 17 communities were selected by the steering committee and invited to participate, and 34 community residents were selected by their communities to be interviewers. Because resident listings in native communities are politically contentious, usually confidential, and not necessarily up to date, the survey sample was drawn from houses randomly selected from a map of each community. The response rate was 81%, showing the strong community support for the survey. (National response rates for the Canadian Community Health Survey are about 85%, excluding residents of aboriginal reserves [Béland et al. 2001].)

Epidemiologic studies can be designed in partnership with communities, and even communities that are hostile to further research can collaborate effectively when they have a chance to influence research objectives and procedures. More details of this study's content can be found on the website of the University of Manitoba's Center for Aboriginal Health Research.

An Example of the Epidemiology of Local Knowledge in Mexico

Following his training in epidemiology at the University of North Carolina (see Chapter 2), medical anthropologist Arthur Rubel became interested in using epidemiologic techniques to study what it means in other cultures to become ill. He picked a condition fairly common in Mexico, *susto*, which has causal explanations and management strategies that would be quite unfamiliar to most biomedical practitioners in the United States. *Susto* is caused by fright or other strong emotion; its victims are thought to lose a vital part of themselves in this process (Rubel et al. 1984). The condition can develop after near-drownings, falls, or other accidents; sightings of snakes; physical threats; and other surprising or stress-laden events. Its victims sleep restlessly and also are "listless, debilitated, depressed, and indifferent to food and to dress and personal hygiene" (Rubel et al. 1984:6). It can be treated through ceremonies designed to identify the event that caused the vital part to depart, and then to return the vital substance to the body.

Rubel's first article on this topic argued that epidemiologic techniques could be used to describe the prevalence and causes of nonbiomedical disease categories (1964). In his later interdisciplinary study (1984), Rubel and colleagues compared the causes, management, and outcomes of *susto* among three distinctly different groups in Mexico. They concluded that people who suffered from *susto* also had relatively high levels of biological disease and tended to die prematurely. But they were careful to point out that *susto* could not be reduced to any single biomedical condition, rather it seemed to indicate a combination of impaired ability to perform critical tasks and the presence of a broad variety of biological diseases. As they put it, people suffering from *susto* were "forced to the sidelines by excessive demands on their adaptive resources" (1984:122). There were differences across the communities in the type of symptoms associated with *susto* and also differences across them in the level of disease burden *susto* posed. These studies by Rubel were important predecessors to the studies of *nervios* and *ataques* mentioned in the first chapter of this book and to many other labels for human suffering that do not fit standard biomedical categories. In short, they show that biomedical definitions need not always form the diagnostic core of epidemiology.

Implications of Popular and Lay Epidemiology for Practice

Epidemiological research is increasingly complex and open to debate both within and outside the discipline. For example, epidemiologists argue against other epidemiologists when policies to limit antibiotic use or reduce smoking are debated. The field's legitimacy as science also is increasingly questioned by other experts as it progresses from description to intervention, and as it shifts its attention from the habits of citizens to the production practices of industries.

People working within the framework of community-controlled epidemiology could argue that community participation in disease surveillance increases the relevance and quality of that science. Those working within the epidemiology of local knowledge could argue that communities draw on multiple sources of expertise outside of biomedical science when establishing what risks matter and what can be done about them. The challenge to both these approaches is that many health risks today are broadly distributed, complex, and hard to measure. Many individuals feel menaced by these risks. But it is not only individuals who feel menaced: industry, entire communities, developers, and governments have disparate and often conflicting interests in measuring disease and risk burdens. A prediction two decades ago about the future of epidemiology in the year 2000 (Rothman 1981) held that epidemiologists would end up debating those risks in the courtroom rather than in the scientific literature. That has happened sometimes, but an equally large challenge to epidemiology is that the public now sees health risks as pervasive but contradictory components of the environment, and it is capable of dismissing them as scientific confusion. Public exposure to epidemiologic findings may not always bring deeper understanding. Such exposure also does not necessarily create public pressure for greater relevance and quality in epidemiologic research.

Epidemiologists measure risks and bring them to public attention, yet this very process causes their authority to be increasingly debated. The *Lancet* editorial asking "Do epidemiologists cause epidemics?" described the dangers resulting when epidemiologic mistakes like improper age standardization and poorly chosen denominators are compounded by the discipline's "popularity with editors, both medical and in the tabloid press" (1993:993). Epidemiology's renown poses benefits and hindrances: many are listening, but errors and overblown claims can be spread as broadly and quickly as well-founded and carefully interpreted results.

Popular and lay epidemiology face different challenges in their efforts to link professionals and nonprofessionals. One major weakness of popular epidemiology is its assumption that citizen participation means citizen adoption of professional concerns and standards. When the public perceives itself as menaced rather than merely at risk and it wants to reduce the threat, it can react in the realms both of science and politics. In the longer term the public can pressure legislators to invest in health research, and in the shorter term it can pressure them to create new programs and special investigations. In an ironic twist, politicians often then transfer the public perception of risk from their political realm back to the scientific realm, by calling for expert reviews and commissions. Expert committees can validate a sense of public menace by finding some statistically, politically, and clinically significant risk factor, or they can dismiss a risk as being indistinguishable from chance. This type of move often buys time for politicians, but it seldom addresses the public's fear (see Nash and Kirsch 1986).

Advocates of lay epidemiology understand this because they are willing to accord legitimacy to popular perceptions that may not be consistent with scientific evidence. But they face their own challenges when they argue that worldviews are legitimate even when they depart from, ignore, or contest biomedical assumptions about disease causation and taxonomy. A large challenge to epidemiology of any type is the ability of interest groups to mobilize politically for change even when most health professionals doubt the evidence, as seen in the United States in the silicone breast implant controversy or concerns about the health risks posed by video display units, high-tension power lines, immunizations, or fluoridated water.

II.   Communicating about Risk, Menace, and Safety

Anthropological Offerings

Anthropologists have spent a fair amount of time analyzing and critiquing epidemiological concepts of risk and perceived risk (DiGiacomo 1999, Gifford 1986, Nations 1986). In an important study of the social impact and cultural meanings of prenatal diagnosis, anthropologist Rayna Rapp interviewed a broad variety of groups involved in developing, collecting, assessing, and deciding what to do with the results of prenatal tests, including pregnant women who accepted or refused the tests, geneticists, genetic counselors, lab technicians, and families of children who have the disabilities revealed by the tests. She explored the language used in counseling sessions, explaining that "positive family histories" meant negative things to counselors, whereas "uneventful" pregnancies indicated no need for further testing.

According to Rapp, the terminology of genetic counseling is played out in a series of "scripts" that convey scientific information, collect and classify patient knowledge, or move back and forth between these in an interaction designed to address patients' concerns (1999:63). Rapp's close analysis of these different objectives helps show how counselors adapt their metaphors and choose levels of technical complexity depending on their assessments of their audience. But Rapp also explores the function of statistics as a "genre of communication" that requires interpretation and shapes client perceptions, a genre that is comfortable and available to educated patients but quite alien and unreal to the uneducated. She writes of a "homegrown sense of statistics" that links personal experience to more general statistical pictures (1999:69). Her analysis reveals the processes through which epidemiologic data become reinterpreted by counselors and their clients.

Epidemiologists are very concerned with the accuracy of their data, but they tend not to be as concerned with the dissemination and interpretation of data subsequent to their scientific reports in journals. Yet diffusion is accompanied by important symbolic transformations: individuals reinterpret scientific reports according to their own experience and systems of meaning. Some compare the abstract risks of getting diabetes or heart disease in the future to the real-life pleasures of eating and drinking today. Others decide to rebuild their home for a third time on the flood plain because they like the view. Still others purchase water filters to reduce their health risk from chemical exposure but ignore the fact that their filters do not screen out the more common and deadly bacterial pathogens that cause diarrheal disease.

Organizations (companies, lobbying groups, governments) repackage and redistribute scientific reports to serve their objectives. Reports of risk and benefit almost invariably improve the commercial or political status of some interest groups while reducing the status of others. It is no wonder, then, that the scientific and legislative battles over the dangers of alcohol abuse, for example, also are expressed as advertising battles containing images of sexy women and injunctions to "drink responsibly" on one side, and images of car wrecks and disfigured teenagers on the other.

Messages about risk can be framed in at least two ways: they can highlight individual (internal) choices about what actions to take or they can highlight external constraints that limit individual freedom to choose health (Frankenberg 1988). Health is often perceived in the United States as personal rather than social (Toumey 1996:78), so American messages about risk tend to highlight individual choice rather than external limits. A glance at some of the popular books designed to help people think about risk shows this bias toward "deciding what's really safe and what's really dangerous in the world around you," which is the subtitle of a book by Ropeik and Gray (2002). The subtitle suggests that risks exist out there in the world, but they can be controlled through individual knowledge and choice.

Risk fills a particular cultural niche in contemporary society. Anthropologists have long said that non-Western cultures explain misfortune partly through magic and witchcraft. Anthropologist E. E. Evans-Pritchard wrote in his classic book *Witchcraft, Oracles and Magic among the Azande* that his African village informants were perfectly capable of explaining that a raised granary collapsed because termites had eaten through the supports (Evans-Pritchard 1937). But witchcraft explained why *that* particular granary collapsed just when *that* particular individual was seated underneath it enjoying the shade. A contemporary social anthropologist suggests that the concept of "risk" plays an equivalent role in post-industrial Western cultures: "where control over one's life has become increasingly viewed as important, the concept of 'risk' is now widely used to explain deviations from the norm, misfortune and frightening events" (Lupton 1999:3).

Anthropologists have argued that risk should be analyzed using ethnographic methods so that it can be tied to particular times, places, and people. In agreement with the quote from Slovic near the beginning of this chapter, they assert that analyses of risk must attend to power and must look at people's involvement in webs of relationships (Caplan 2000:26–27). One example of this is a study of AIDS in northern Tanzania that argues that epidemiologic research on HIV risk focuses on easily definable components of sexual behavior like number of partners and categories of relationship (Setel 1999). Standard HIV research misses many complex and changing forms of partnership, duration of spousal separation, and the social conditions under which some types of relationships are sustained and others unsupported – information critical to understanding why people are exposed to HIV infection (Setel 1999:83–86). This is an example of looking at the "risk factors behind the risk factors" that was described in Chapter 6.

Lay epidemiology itself is the subject of new research. Some are asking how policy debates around epidemiologic controversies represent and include the voices and claims of non-experts (e.g., Moffatt et al. 2000).

This work explores what might be done to increase participation and influence of non-experts in such debates. Others ask how different groups use epidemiologic data in conversation, as guides to daily behavior, and as rationales for self-defined states of health or illness. Some have done content analyses of epidemiologic news as reported in the mass media (e.g., Greenberg and Wartenberg 1990). When Bartlett et al. undertook such a study of research published in two British medical journals and two popular newspapers, they discovered that randomized clinical trial designs and results considered to be "bad news" were less likely to be published in newspapers, as was any kind of research coming from developing countries (2002). Much more needs to be known about how public health data of all kinds are disseminated and circulated within populations, and how different publics perceive epidemiology and epidemiologic data. How does the power and public image of epidemiology vary between the United States and European nations, or among Mexico, Brazil, Japan, and Germany? Samples of the medical literature taken from different countries show varying levels of attention paid to epidemiologic data (Takahashi et al. 2001).

How Epidemiologists Create Epidemics and Other Reactions

Although epidemiologists might wonder at the hubris of the *Lancet* asking if they cause epidemics, anthropologists would readily reply, "Why, of course they do!" Most epidemiologists would recoil from what anthropologists find quite acceptable: that the public's epidemiologic understanding goes beyond what it knows about epidemiologic method. This public understanding encompasses what epidemiology is used for and whether people find it personally relevant. Anthropologists know that epidemiology produces metaphors even as it produces knowledge about disease causation and prevention. These metaphors include qualities like "safe" sex and "good" cholesterol, but they also include confusing contradictions between risks and benefits of consuming specific foods. Contradictory information puts people in the difficult bind of choosing between whether to drink red wine to reduce the risk of heart disease or to avoid red wine to reduce the risk of liver disease. Conflicting data about fat and heart disease create consumer dilemmas about whether to purchase butter, margarine, or a product cleverly labeled to capitalize on these contradictions, called "I Can't Believe It's Not Butter," available in regular and "light" versions. Small protective effects of oatmeal on heart disease or fiber on colorectal cancers are rapidly translated into commercial claims that eating Brand X cereal with lots of added fiber is good for one's health.

Equivalent rifts exist between the number of cases of some diseases and their perceived menace. The real number of cases of disease that are major news items such as anthrax, West Nile virus, and Ebola virus is much smaller than the total of deaths from the major killers like lung cancer and heart disease in industrialized settings, and childhood infectious diseases, malaria, and AIDS in developing countries. In sum, epidemiology is known and remembered by the public far more for its claims and metaphors than for its specific data about relative risk and incidence rates.

How do epidemiologists create epidemics? Epidemiologists create perceptions of risk in their audiences at least partly by how they describe disease outcomes. For example, when asked to choose between two cancer therapies, one group was given data on probability of surviving, the other on probability of dying (McNeil et al. 1982:1259). When the choice was phrased in terms of probability of surviving, 18% chose radiation therapy over surgery; when phrased in terms of dying, 44% chose radiation therapy over surgery. The percentages changed in similar fashion when physicians answered, with 16% choosing radiation therapy over surgery when outcomes were expressed as probability of surviving, and 50% when expressed as probability of dying. It appears that these audiences paid attention to risk phrased as hope rather than despair.

Physicians also react differently to risk when it is presented as a dilemma facing an individual patient compared with the same dilemma facing an entire group. Rudelmeier and Tversky (1990) presented physicians with a series of paired clinical scenarios in which one version asked how a single patient should be treated, and the other version asked how a group of comparable patients should be treated. They reported that "physicians give more weight to the personal concerns of patients when considering them as individuals and more weight to general criteria of effectiveness when considering them as a group" (1990:1163). This very likely means that epidemiologic data meant to guide clinical practice will have more impact on physicians when described in terms of an individual case than in terms of a group tendency.

Psychological studies of the interpretation of risk, and perception of risk as high or low, reveal some consistent differences across groups. For example, "White" males consistently perceive the risks of potentially hazardous activities as lower than both "White" women and than "non-Whites" of both sexes (Slovic 1997:73). Age also makes a difference in how people perceive risk. Young people aged 14 to 22 try smoking primarily because they feel it will relax them and help them feel good. This is even more important than their perception about the dangers of smoking – in fact "apart from their feelings toward smoking, there is no evidence that recognition of risks deters young people from trying smoking or progressing toward a smoking habit" (Romer and Jamieson 2001b:70–71). Adults, on the other hand, reduce their smoking more as their perception of its danger increases (*Ibid.*:71). Given these types of systematic differences, it is fair to conclude that risk perception is culturally shaped rather than idiosyncratic.

In fact, most evaluations of hazard perceptions in the United States find they can be displayed in two basic dimensions: one axis corresponds to whether they are known (observable, known to those exposed, of immediate effect, known to science) or not, and the other axis corresponds to whether they are dreaded (uncontrollable, globally catastrophic, fatal, involuntary) or not. For example, the hazards of radioactive waste are unknown and dreaded, nuclear weapons hazards are known and dreaded; bicycle hazards are known and not dreaded, and water fluoridation hazards are unknown and dreaded (Slovic 1987). Studies comparing these perceptions across Poland, the United States, Hungary, and Norway found essentially the same dimensions used in each country (Goszczynska et al. 1991). As yet, however, there is little other comparative data available about perceptions of risk in other sites.

III.   A Few Lessons and Opportunities

Prior chapters emphasized the importance of risk and communication even as they attended to issues of definitions, measurements, and intervention designs. This one looked at three different aspects of risk: first, how epidemiologists pay attention to public efforts to measure their own health risks (popular epidemiology); second, how epidemiologic methods can be used to study suffering and disease entities that may not be defined according to biomedical theories (lay epidemiology); and third, how epidemiologists and the general public exchange information about risk, and what happens to scientific claims about probability and likelihood as they get transmitted from producers to consumers.

The lessons and opportunities offered by popular and lay epidemiology are linked to how risk is constructed and communicated. The seductive power of numbers and graphics can divert researchers' and readers' attention away from the content of messages and toward their form (Tufte 1983). Graphical displays may be the only way to reach some audiences (Edwards et al. 2002), but others find them unintelligible or superfluous or distracting (Fortin et al. 2001). The pioneering work of Robert Chambers and others can be taken further into the domain of health, asking how participatory mapping techniques can better represent neighborhood disease burden and exploring how graphical displays and other methods can convey epidemiologic statistics to poorly educated or even illiterate populations. These are ways to expand the tools available for use in popular epidemiology. Disease mapping by community residents and participatory mapping strategies suggest that there are other opportunities to employ graphic and geographic methods to bring researchers and community members closer together. Popular and lay epidemiology are both experiments in creating more sensitive and profound displays of the social and cultural patternings of disease across the landscape. They both describe risk as a collective rather than individual phenomenon.

Epidemiologic results go through many transformations between their production as statistics, publication and circulation as scientific papers, popularization through mass media, and absorption by individual citizens. Journalists and the general public both rapidly interpret new data. These interpretations draw on fundamental beliefs about what types of activities are dangerous and what levels of risk are acceptable. As health scientists in all disciplines become more accustomed to dealing with a broad range of reactions from diverse audiences, they are acquiring skills in media relations and in writing for the public. They are especially well served by emphasizing the tentative nature of their results, calling for confirmation from other sources and taking care not to overinterpret their data when transforming statistical estimates of risk into concrete recommendations for treatment or behavioral change.

FOR FURTHER READING

Chambers R. 1997. *Whose Reality Counts? Putting the First Last.* London: Intermediate Technology Publications.
Douglas M. 1992. *Risk and Blame: Essays in Cultural Theory.* New York: Routledge.
Slovic P. 1987. Perception of risk. *Science* 236:280–285.
Tufte E. R. 1990. *Envisioning Information.* Chesire, CT: Graphics Press.

8   Conclusion

Diseases are strangely intimate disorders, eliciting private sensations and personal emotions. They also are achingly public experiences, especially frightening when counting makes them visible. Descriptions of disease often move back and forth between textual and statistical portrayals, between pain and hope in individuals, and between cancer rates or life expectancy in populations. For example, the public was put on notice by a *Time* magazine cover in 1998 that blared: "THE KILLER GERM. It's turning up everywhere: in your water, your food, the pool. How to protect yourself from E. Coli." But the article began with this sentence: "Tammy Lowery couldn't see the blood vessels rupturing in her gut, but the way she was feeling, she didn't have to." This sensationalized introduction mixes general menace ("turning up everywhere") with personal exposure ("your water, your food"), and a specific person (Tammy). Journalistic accounts like this often describe sick individuals as a hook to draw their readers' attention and increase their interest; they present disease statistics to help their audience feel – and perhaps also understand – the magnitude of a health problem.

Health researchers have been far more reluctant than journalists to mix stories about sick individuals with statistics about disease patterns. Researchers tend to communicate within their own disciplines more than with others, and most have little or nothing to do with the general public. They get trained in, and rely on, a limited number of forms of knowledge exchange. This can be detrimental when they seek interdisciplinary or public conversations, for in these exchanges case histories can be dismissed as "mere anecdote," just as readily as statistics can be dismissed as "faceless numbers." Researchers and practitioners in population health can combine individual case reports and statistical accounts without distorting either one; learning how to do this is difficult, but it can be effective.

Do I mean that researchers need to become journalists? No. Journalism is a structured way to convert news and information into a compelling story, whereas research is a structured and systematic way to seek knowledge through specified methods. Knowledge is useless if not communicated, but it is also useless if not understood. And the greatest health problems confronting the world today, like AIDS, tuberculosis, childhood infections, lung cancer, heart disease, and stroke, require solutions at least partly based on knowledge from multiple cooperating disciplines. The limited ability to communicate across disciplines, and to reach beyond disciplines to the general public, is a substantial part of the challenge facing those trying to reduce and prevent global health problems.

Society and culture are fixed in the very center of the epidemiologic categories of person, place, and time. If these categories were used to explain the origins of the E. coli epidemic they would have to take account of personal decisions, pathogen mutations, water quality, and corporate and government policies. Diseases have "natural" and "sociocultural" histories, which must be interwoven if we are to use the origins of disease as clues to their treatment and prevention.

The contrast between Tammy's gut and an E. coli epidemic emphasizes the complementarity between textual and statistical portrayals of disease. Disease portraits are built from personal decisions as well as virulence and incidence rates. But of course the relationships between text and statistics and between personal risk and general menace are more complicated than that. Textual and statistical portrayals each are constructed from many layers of data. Standard methods of collecting epidemiologic data also are subject to local influence, either through research participants' behavior and reactions or through researchers' own unexamined assumptions about measurement. Public health interventions themselves create or minimize perceptions of risk and incite or quell responses. So do textual, numerical, graphical, and geographical "pictures" of disease and risk. The polarized difference between statistical and textual descriptions is more complex than it may first appear.

The narrative in this book provides many examples of collaborative projects drawing on theories and methods from both anthropology and epidemiology. Interdisciplinary studies are emerging from teams of researchers in many places, trained in many disciplines and able to communicate across them. But any researcher working in one discipline should be able to use the methods and theories from another, as long as they understand and use them well. An epidemiologist can include an ethnographic component to explore motivations for behavior change, and an anthropologist can mount a case-control study to examine the causes of a folk illness. The types of cross-cutting examples described in this book have been undertaken by one person borrowing from both disciplines, individuals sharing across disciplines, and groups creating new disciplines.

After the anthrax outbreaks in the United States in 2001, a *New Yorker* magazine cartoon portrayed a society woman introducing "her epidemiologist" to her guests at a fashionable cocktail party. Epidemiologists are not yet quite this popular, but the results of their research have surely become indispensable. And recent trends toward "evidence-based medicine" make epidemiology more popular in clinical journals than ever before. Fascinating debates are being played out as clinicians try to evaluate their own individual decisions and their own individual training experiences compared with those recommended in RCTs. Much as the general public is buffeted by conflicting news reports about high-risk foods or preventive health behaviors, buffeted also are medical educators divided about whether their new curricular experiments can be tested in controlled trials (Prideaux 2002) and psychiatrists concerned that RCTs be interpreted along with clinical expertise about a specific individual (Williams and Garner 2002). What measurements, and what techniques, produce knowledge that is considered to be valid? These, also, are cultural questions, and their answers change over time.

I.   Epidemiology, Proof and Judgment

"Naturally," Dr. Greenberg said, "it would have been nice to know for a fact that the old boys all sat at a certain table and that all of them put about a spoonful of salt from that particular shaker on their oatmeal, but it wasn't essential. I was morally certain that they had. There just wasn't any other explanation." (Roueché 1947 [1980]:1–12).

Berton Roueché, writer for three decades of the Annals of Medicine column for *The New Yorker* magazine, specialized in dramatizing the disease outbreak investigations undertaken by state Public Health Departments and the Communicable Disease Center in Atlanta (forerunner of today's Centers for Disease Control and Prevention). Part detective and part storyteller, Roueché popularized epidemiology for two generations of *New Yorker* readers, showing how epidemiologists traced the causes of small outbreaks of schistosomiasis, trichinosis, anthrax, histoplasmosis, tularemia, and other communicable diseases and conditions rarely seen in the United States. How epidemiologists put evidence together, and what stories are told about that process, are other important parts of the relationship between personal risk and general menace.

Roueché used the strange case of 11 blue men to illustrate how epidemiology can solve mysteries. In 1944, 11 elderly vagrant men in New York City were brought to area hospitals, severely ill and cyanotic (skyblue). One died. An epidemiologic investigation showed that the men were all sickened by a perplexing case of food-poisoning in which they became ill within 30 minutes of eating oatmeal at the same restaurant. The causal agent was sodium nitr*ite*, a dangerous chemical substituted in small quantities during the war for the more benign meat preservative sodium nitr*ate*. Sodium nitrite from a large can on a high shelf in the kitchen was mistakenly used as salt to flavor a vat of oatmeal, and it was mistakenly used to top up one salt shaker at one table in the restaurant. Those who ate the oatmeal alone did not receive a nitrite dose large enough to cause symptoms, so epidemiologists concluded that those who got sick must have flavored their breakfast with the adulterated salt.

The case also shows the role of human values and judgment in the science and practice of epidemiology. The 11 men were all known to have eaten the oatmeal, but all were discharged from the hospital before they could be asked whether they had used extra salt. The epidemiologist used the pattern of the illness, fieldwork in the restaurant, and tests in the laboratory, to infer the behavioral steps intervening between susceptibility and sickness. He deduced the causal pathway from the overall pattern of the illness. There is some paradox in this deduction: the epidemiologist claims to be "morally certain" that he has figured out the causal chain, even in the absence of critical data. The phrase "moral certainty" is, on one hand, a nineteenth-century construction meaning "proof beyond a reasonable doubt." To be morally certain means to have decided on the basis of reason rather than demonstration. In epidemiology that reason is usually brought to bear on statistical summaries of data. Probabilities are calculated of how likely it would be that a particular distribution of lung cancer between smokers and nonsmokers would occur by chance alone. But is this the same as proof of causation? Tobacco companies argued successfully for decades that it was not. The competition between the epidemiologist's moral certainty and the public's desire for demonstration is a fundamental challenge for epidemiology, sometimes interfering with the ability of the discipline to establish clear proof and to communicate well with the public.

This contemporary challenge exists partly because epidemiology has been so successful in discovering the big single risks for the biggest health problems. But the era of discoveries of large risks is about over: only a limited number of substances or actions are so injurious that they cause differences at the magnitude of the 16-fold difference in lung cancer rates between smokers and nonsmokers. Most health risks explored today are multifactorial. When found, risk ratios are more on the order of 2- or 3-fold than 10- or 16-fold (Taubes 1995). Differences smaller than this can potentially be explained away by design and analysis problems, so fewer epidemiologic findings meet with even grudging acceptance.

There are more epidemiologists than ever, making a bigger deal about smaller risks.

If the big risks have been found, however, this does not mean epidemiology has been equally successful at turning those discoveries into effective therapies and policies. The struggle today is to figure out how to turn epidemiologic findings into recommendations for human behavior. Boldness and humility both are important virtues in this task.

II.   Conclusions about Defining Disciplines: Defended Border versus Semi-permeable Membrane

Many successful and innovative interdisciplinary projects have taken place over the past century that describe and/or attempt to improve the health of populations. Anthropologists' involvement with epidemiologists is supported at the beginning of the twenty-first century by extensive U.S. and international funding for chronic health risks, infectious diseases, and international themes related to the survival of children and adults. Contributors to the American Anthropological Association's newsletter have recommended that introductory and advanced epidemiology should form part of a core curriculum for graduate medical anthropology students (American Anthropological Association 1993, 1994). The list of anthropologists who have called for such collaboration is long and growing (for references see Trostle and Sommerfeld 1996). Whereas 19 anthropologists were employed in 1996 in Atlanta at the Centers for Disease Control and Prevention the number in 2001 was closer to 43 (J. Carey, personal communication, 2001). If not yet commonplace, collaboration between medical anthropologists and epidemiologists is certainly increasing.

This book shows that many interdisciplinary projects are taking place between anthropologists and epidemiologists, and it argues that disciplinary attempts to maintain exclusive control over knowledge domains can be counterproductive. Each chapter offers a route to mutual exchange, a way of thinking about disciplinary boundaries as semi-permeable membranes rather than defended borders. The historical review shows the legitimacy of projects joining anthropology with epidemiology: many have studied the causal role society and culture play in human health, and successful interdisciplinary programs have been created over the past seven decades linking anthropology and epidemiology to patient care. How questions are constructed and relevant variables defined is another pathway to collaboration. Although the categories of person, place, and time now seem almost pedestrian in epidemiological studies, this book gives them new life. Some of the more productive areas for interdisciplinary study focus on how these categories overlap, such as how aspects of person and place merge in studies of place-based networks, how person and time coexist in research linking identity and health status, and how place and time intersect in studies showing how context influences behavior and health. Human behavior is contingent. Context influences people's activities, their health risks, and the outcomes of their diseases.

Data collection itself is another fruitful area for joint projects between anthropologists and epidemiologists. Looking at data collection as a process of social exchange allows a novel kind of attention to be paid to the influence of society and culture on health. This influence can be seen in how measurement tools are developed and chosen as well as in the reactions of participants to being measured. Research designs themselves are becoming more complex and are beginning to connect disease processes across molecular, physiological, familial, community, and socioeconomic levels. Public health interventions at the level of communities are another example of contemporary complex designs. They are doubly valuable because they can at once show which behavior strategies can succeed, and they can reveal how communities are put together. Complex designs require contributions from many disciplines, but effective contributions come from knowing what other colleagues need as well as what they value. A fundamental understanding of other disciplines' research designs and data collection methods is critical for successful collaboration.

Epidemiologists and anthropologists are exploring how to involve the public in their collaborative projects and how to use their disciplinary skills to address public concerns. These challenges offer many new opportunities for research and for new forms of communication. The presence and importance of graphical and geographical representations of risk are likely to continue to grow. But they will supplement rather than replace the power of combining textual with numerical displays.

"Cultural epidemiology" forms an important parallel to "social epidemiology." This book argues that epidemiology is a cultural practice, although often it is unrecognized as such. Variables are defined and measured, results quantified, analyses disseminated, and policies developed, all with specific cultural assumptions behind them. Cultural epidemiology reveals the ways in which measurement, causal thinking, and intervention design are all influenced by belief and habit in addition to deduction and rational decision-making.

Cultural epidemiology also describes how group health patterns are built out of what appear to be individual decisions. There are clear cultural influences on ideas as diverse as whether pills are more powerful than injections, when and where a person should be allowed to smoke, and how much physical activity a person should have in a day. These powerful ideas, labeled "values," guide behavior that directly changes human health. Summed across thousands of people, decisions like these yield symptom profiles, incidence rates, and case fatality rates.

But culture is not just a realm of ideas and personal decisions. It is also a set of rankings of human classifications like skin color or religion or caste, which influence the "types" of people or groups that have ready access to resources. And it is a set of public decisions about how much money should be invested in hospitals versus weapons, what kinds of health problems constitute emergencies, and even what kinds of suffering and complaints can be resolved. Questioning these decisions is the biggest challenge in the study of epidemiology and culture.

References

Abramson J. H. and Z. H. Abramson. 1999. *Survey Methods in Community Medicine: Epidemiological Studies, Programme Evaluation, Clinical Trials.* Edinburgh: Churchill Livingstone.

_____. 2001. *Making Sense of Data: A Self-Instruction Manual on the Interpretation of Epidemiologic Data.* Oxford: Oxford University Press.

Ackerknecht E. H. 1948. Anticontagionism between 1821 and 1867. *Bulletin of the History of Medicine* 22:562–593.

_____. 1953. *Rudolf Virchow: Doctor, Statesman, Anthropologist.* Madison: University of Wisconsin Press.

_____. 1967. *Medicine at the Paris Hospital, 1794–1848.* Baltimore: The Johns Hopkins University Press.

Adair J. and K. W. Deuschle. 1970. *The People's Health: Medicine and Anthropology in a Navajo Community.* New York: Appleton-Century-Crofts.

Agar M. 1996. Recasting the "ethno" in "epidemiology." *Medical Anthropology* 16:391–403.

Ahdieh L. and R. A. Hahn. 1996. Use of the terms "race," "ethnicity," and "national origins": a review of articles in the American Journal of Public Health, 1980–1989. *Ethnicity and Health* 1:95–98.

Almeida Filho N. 1992. *Epidemiología sin números.* (Epidemiology without Numbers.) Washington, DC: Pan American Health Organization.

American Anthropological Association. *Anthropology Newsletter.* May 1993, pp. 15–16; September 1993, pp. 41–42; and April 1994, pp. 31–32.

Anderson M. R. and S. Moscou. 1998. Race and ethnicity in research on infant mortality. *Family Medicine* 30:224–227.

Armelagos G. J. and A. H. Goodman. 1998. Race, Racism, and Anthropology. In *Building a New Biocultural Synthesis: Political-Economic Perspectives on Human Biology.* A. H. Goodman and T. L. Leatherman, eds. Pp. 359–377. Ann Arbor: University of Michigan Press.

Asad T. 1994. Ethnographic representation, statistics, and modern power. *Social Research* 61:55–88.

Atrostic B. K., N. Bates, G. Burt, A. Silberstein, and F. Winters. 1999. Nonresponse in federal household surveys: new measures and new insights. Paper presented at the International Conference on Survey Nonresponse, Portland, Oregon, October 1999. Available online at: http://www.jpsm.umd.edu/icsn/papers/atrostic.htm#_ftn1. Accessed October 2001.

Audy J. R. 1958. Medical ecology in relation to geography. *British Journal of Clinical Practice* 12:102–110.

Austin H., H. A. Hill, D. Flanders, and R. S. Greenberg. 1994. Nonparticipation of eligible controls may bias results. Limitations in the application of case-control methodology. *Epidemiologic Reviews* 16:65–76.

Baer H., M. Singer, and I. Susser. 1997. *Medical Anthropology and the World System*. New York: Greenwood.

Bartlett C., J. Sterne, and M. Egger. 2002. What is newsworthy? Longitudinal study of the reporting of medical research in two British newspapers. *British Medical Journal* 325:81–84.

Beals B. 1953. Acculturation. In *Anthropology Today*. A. L. Kroeber, ed. Pp. 621–641. Chicago: University of Chicago Press.

Béhague D. P., C. G. Victora, and F. C. Barros. 2002. Consumer demand for caesarean sections in Brazil: informed decision making, patient choice, or social inequality? A population based birth cohort study linking ethnographic and epidemiological methods. *British Medical Journal* 324:942–947.

Béland Y., J. Dufour, and M. Hamel. 2001. Preventing non-response in the Canadian Health Survey. Proceedings of Statistics Canada's Symposium 2001, Achieving Data Quality in a Statistical Agency. Catalogue No.: 11-522-XIE, Ottawa, September 2002. Available online at: http://www.statcan.ca/english/conferences/symposium2002/session9/s9d.pdf. Accessed April 2003.

Bell C. M. and D. A. Redelmeier. 2001. Mortality among patients admitted to hospitals on weekends as compared with weekdays. *New England Journal of Medicine* 345:663–668.

Bentley M. E. 1992. Household behaviors in the management of diarrhea and their relevance for persistent diarrhea. *Acta Paediatrica* 381 (Suppl):49–54.

Beran R. G., J. Michelazzi, L. Hall, P. Tsimnadis, and S. Loh. 1985. False-negative response rate in epidemiologic studies to define prevalence ratios of epilepsy. *Neuroepidemiology* 4:82–85.

Berkman L. F. and S. L. Syme. 1979. Social networks, host resistance, and mortality: a nine-year follow-up of Alameda County residents. *American Journal of Epidemiology* 109:186–204.

Berkman L. F. and I. Kawachi, eds. 2000. *Social Epidemiology*. Oxford: Oxford University Press.

Berney L. R. and D. B. Lane. 1997. Collecting retrospective data: accuracy of recall after 50 years judged against historical records. *Social Science and Medicine* 45:1519–1525.

Bewell A. 1999. *Romanticism and Colonial Disease*. Baltimore: The Johns Hopkins University Press.

Black N. 1994. Why we need qualitative research. *Journal of Epidemiology and Community Health* 48:425–426.

Blalock H. M. 1968. The Measurement Problem: A Gap between the Languages of Theory and Research. In *Methodology in Social Research*. H. M. Blalock and A. B. Blalock, eds. Pp. 5–27. New York: McGraw-Hill.

———. 1990. Auxiliary Measurement Theories Revisited. In *Operationalization and Research Strategy*. J. J. DeJong-Gierveld and J. Hox, eds. Pp. 33–48. Amsterdam: Swets and Zeitlinger.

Blankenship K. M., S. J. Bray, and M. H. Merson. 2000. Structural interventions in public health. *AIDS* 14 (Suppl 1):S11–S21.

Blumenthal D., E. G. Campbell, M. S. Anderson, N. Causino, and K. S. Louis. 1997. Withholding research results in academic life science: evidence from a national survey of faculty. *Journal of the American Medical Association* 277:1224–1228.

Boerma J. T., R. E. Black, A. E. Sommerfelt, S. O. Rutstein, and G. T. Bicego. 1991. Accuracy and completeness of mothers' recall of diarrhoea occurrence in pre-school children in demographic and health surveys. *International Journal of Epidemiology* 20:1073–1080.

Borroto R. J. and R. Martinez Piedra. 2000. Geographical patterns of cholera in Mexico, 1991–1996. *International Journal of Epidemiology* 29:764–772.

Bourgois P. 1999. Theory, method, and power in drug and HIV-prevention research: a participant-observer's critique. *Substance Use and Misuse* 34:2155–2172.

———. 2002. Anthropology and epidemiology on drugs: the challenges of cross-methodological and theoretical dialogue. *International Journal of Drug Policy* 13:259–269.

Breilh J. 1994. Nuevos Conceptos y Técnicas de Investigación [New Research Concepts and Techniques]. Serie: "Epidemiología Crítica [Series: Critical Epidemiology]," No. 3. Quito, Ecuador: Centro de Estudios y Asesoría en Salud.

Brewster K. L. 1994. Neighborhood context and the transition to sexual activity among young black women. *Demography* 31:603–614.

Briggs C. L. 1999. Lessons in the time of cholera. In Infectious Diseases and Social Inequality in Latin America: From Hemispheric Insecurity to Global Cooperation. Latin American Program, Working Paper Series no. 239. Pp. 1–30. Washington, DC: Woodrow Wilson International Center for Scholars.

Briggs C. L. and C. Mantini-Briggs. 2003. *Stories in the Time of Cholera.* Berkeley: University of California Press.

Brooks-Gunn J., P. Duncan, P. K. Klebanov, and N. Sealand. 1993. Do neighborhoods influence child and adolescent development? *American Journal of Sociology* 99:353–395.

Brown P. 1992. Popular epidemiology and toxic waste contamination: lay and professional ways of knowing. *Journal of Health and Social Behavior* 33:267–281.

Brown P., E. J. Mikkelsen, and J. Harr. 1990. *No Safe Place: Toxic Waste, Leukemia, and Community Action.* Berkeley: University of California Press.

Buck A. A., R. I. Anderson, K. Kawata, R. A. Ward, T. T. Sasaki, and F. M. Amin. 1972. *Health and Disease in Rural Afghanistan.* Baltimore: York Press.

Buck A. A., R. I. Anderson, T. T. Sasaki, and K. Kawata. 1970. *Health and Disease in Chad: Epidemiology, Culture, and Environment in Five Villages.* Baltimore: The Johns Hopkins University Press.

Buck A. A., T. T. Sasaki, and R. I. Anderson. 1968. *Health and Disease in Four Peruvian Villages: Contrasts in Epidemiology.* Baltimore: The Johns Hopkins University Press.

Burrage H. 1987. Epidemiology and community health: a strained connection? *Social Science and Medicine* 25:895–903.

Caplan P. 2000. Introduction: Risk Revisited. In *Risk Revisited*. P. Caplan, ed. Pp. 1–28. London: Pluto Press.

Casper M. 1997. Feminist politics and fetal surgery: adventures of a research cowgirl on the reproductive frontier. *Feminist Studies* 23:232–263.

Cassel J. C. 1955. A Comprehensive Health Program among South African Zulus. In *Health, Culture, and Community. Case Studies of Public Reactions to Health Programs*. B. D. Paul, ed. Pp. 15–41. New York: Russell Sage Foundation.

———. 1962. Cultural Factors in the Interpretation of Illness. A Case Study. In *A Practice of Social Medicine*. S. L. Kark and G. W. Steuart, eds. Pp. 238–244. Edinburgh: E. & S. Livingstone.

———. 1964. Social science theory as a source of hypotheses in epidemiological research. *American Journal of Public Health* 54:1482–1488.

———. 1976. The contribution of the social environment to host resistance. *American Journal of Epidemiology* 104:107–123.

Cassel J. C. and H. A. Tyroler. 1961. Epidemiological studies of culture change I: health status and recency of industrialization. *Archives of Environmental Health* 3:25–33.

Cassel J. C., R. C. Patrick Jr., and C. D. Jenkins. 1960. Epidemiologic analysis of the health implications of culture change. A conceptual model. *Annals of the New York Academy of Sciences* 84:938–949.

Caudill W. 1953. Applied Anthropology in Medicine. In *Anthropology Today*. A. L. Kroeber, ed. Pp.771–806. Chicago: University of Chicago Press.

Centers for Disease Control and Prevention. 1992. *Principles of Epidemiology*. 2nd edition. Self-Study Course 3030-G. Atlanta: Centers for Disease Control.

———. 1993. Monthly Vital Statistics Report 42, no. 2(S), July 8. Available online at: http://www.cdc.gov/nchs/data/mvsr/supp/mvsr42_2sjulacc.pdf. Accessed December 2001.

———. 2003. *Cholera: Technical Information*. Division of Bacterial and Mycotic Diseases. Available online at: http://www.cdc.gov/ncidod/dbmd/diseaseinfo/cholera_t.htm. Accessed June 2004.

Chambers R. 1997. What Works and Why? In *Whose Reality Counts? Putting the First Last*. Pp. 130–161. London: Intermediate Technology Publications.

Chen K. H. and G. F. Murray. 1976. Truths and Untruths in Village Haiti: An Experiment in Third World Survey Research. In *Culture, Natality and Family Planning*. J. F. Marshall and S. Polgar, eds. Pp. 241–262. Chapel Hill: University of North Carolina Press.

Chiahemen J. 1995. It is much more frightening...the spread has begun. *The Independent* (London) May 14:1.

Chrisman N. J. 1977. The health seeking process: an approach to the natural history of illness. *Culture, Medicine and Psychiatry* 1:351–377.

Cohen M. N. 1989. *Health and the Rise of Civilization*. New Haven, CT: Yale University Press.

Coimbra C. Jr. and J. Trostle, eds. 2004. *Abordagens Antropológicas em Epidemiologia* [Anthropological Approaches to Epidemiology]. Rio de Janeiro: Editora Fiocruz.

Corbett K. K. 2001. Susceptibility of youth to tobacco: a social ecological framework for prevention. *Respiration Physiology* 128:103–118.

Cosminsky S., M. Mhloyi, and D. Ewbank. 1993. Child feeding practices in a rural area of Zimbabwe. *Social Science and Medicine* 36:937–947.

Crane J. 1991. The epidemic theory of ghettos and neighborhood effects on dropping out and teenage childbearing. *American Journal of Sociology* 96:1226–1259.

Creamer G., N. León, M. Kenber, P. Samaniego, and G. Buchholz. 1999. Efficiency of hospital cholera treatment in Ecuador. *Revista Panamericana de Salud Publica* 5:77–87.

Cueto M. 1997. *El Regreso de las Epidemias: Salud y Sociedad en el Perú del Siglo XX* [The Return of Epidemics: Health and Society in Twentieth-Century Peru]. Lima: Instituto de Estudios Peruanos.

Davey Smith G. and E. Susser. 2002. Zena Stein, Mervyn Susser, and epidemiology: observation, causation and action. *International Journal of Epidemiology* 31:34–37.

Davey Smith G., M. J. Shipley, and G. Rose. 1990. Magnitude and causes of socioeconomic differentials in mortality: further evidence from the Whitehall Study. *Journal of Epidemiology and Community Health* 44:265–270.

Davidoff F., C. D. DeAngelis, J. M. Drazen, M. G. Nicholls, J. Hoey, L. Hojgaard, R. Horton, S. Kotzin, M. Nylenna, A. J. Overbeke, H. C. Sox, M. B. Van Der Weyden, and M. S. Wilkes. 2001. Sponsorship, authorship, and accountability. *New England Journal of Medicine* 345:825–826.

Dawson R. J. M. 1995. The "unusual episode" data revisited. *Journal of Statistics Education* 3. Available online at: http://www.stat.unipg.it/ncsu/info/jse/v3n3/datasets.dawson.html. Accessed March 2001.

Day S. J. and D. G. Altman. 2000. Blinding in clinical trials and other studies. *British Medical Journal* 321:504.

Denberg T., M. Welch, and M. D. Feldman. 2003. Cross-cultural communication. In *Behavioral Medicine in Primary Care*. M. D. Feldman and J. F. Christensen, eds. Pp. 103–113. New York: McGraw-Hill.

DiGiacomo S. 1999. Can there be a "cultural epidemiology?" *Medical Anthropology Quarterly* 13:436–457.

Donkin A., Y. H. Lee, and B. Toson. 2002. Implications of changes in the U.K. social and occupational classifications in 2001 for vital statistics. The effect of three innovations in the reporting of vital statistics. *Population Trends* 107:23–29. Available online at: http://www.statistics.gov.uk/articles/population_trends/sococclassifications_pt107.pdf. Accessed May 2004.

Donovan J., N. Mills, M. Smith, L. Brindle, A. Jacoby, T. Peters, S. Frankel, D. Neal, F. Hamdy, and P. Little. 2002. Improving design and conduct of randomised trials by embedding them in qualitative research: ProtecT (prostate testing for cancer and treatment) study. *British Medical Journal* 325:766–770.

Douglas M. 1992. *Risk and Blame: Essays in Cultural Theory.* London: Routledge.

Downey A. M., S. J. Virgilio, D. C. Serpas, T. A. Nicklas, M. L. Arbeit, and G. S. Berenson. 1988. "Heart Smart" – a staff development model for a school-based cardiovascular health intervention. *Health Education* 19:64–71.

Dressler W. W. 1999. Modernization, stress, and blood pressure: new directions in research. *Human Biology* 71:583–605.

Dressler W. W., J. E. Dos Santos, and M. C. Balieiro. 1996. Studying diversity and sharing in culture: an example of lifestyle in Brazil. *Journal of Anthropological Research* 52:331–353.

Dressler W. W., M. C. Balieiro, and J. E. Dos Santos. 1997. The cultural construction of social support in Brazil: associations with health outcomes. *Culture, Medicine and Psychiatry* 21:303–335.

Dunn F. L. 1979. Behavioral aspects of the control of parasitic diseases. *Bulletin of the World Health Organization* 57:499–512.

Dunn F. L. and C. R. Janes. 1986. Introduction: medical anthropology and epidemiology. In *Anthropology and Epidemiology: Interdisciplinary Approaches to the Study of Health and Disease.* C. R. Janes, R. Stall, and S. Gifford, eds. Pp. 3–34. Dordrecht, The Netherlands: Reidel.

Durkheim E. 1951 [1897]. *Suicide: A Study in Sociology.* Rev. edition. (1st French ed., 1897.) J. A. Spaulding and G. Simpson, trans. Glencoe, IL: The Free Press.

Edwards A. 2003. Communicating risks. *British Medical Journal* 327:691–692.

Edwards A., G. Elwyn, and A. Mulley. 2002. Explaining risks: turning numeric data into meaningful pictures. *British Medical Journal* 324:827–830.

Ene-Obong H. N., C. U. Iroegbu, and A. C. Uwaegbute. 2000. Perceived causes and management of diarrhoea in young children by market women in Enugu State, Nigeria. *Journal of Health, Population and Nutrition* 18:97–102.

Engle P. L. and J. B. Lumpkin. 1992. How accurate are time-use reports – effects of cognitive enhancement and cultural-differences on recall accuracy. *Applied Cognitive Psychology* 6:141–159.

Epstein P. R. 1992. Cholera and the environment: an introduction to climate change. Unpublished manuscript. Boston: Harvard Medical School.

Ernster V., N. Kaufman, M. Nichter, J. Samet, and S. Y. Yoon. 2000. Women and tobacco: moving from policy to action. *Bulletin of the World Health Organization* 78:891–901.

Evans-Pritchard E. E. 1937. *Witchcraft, Oracles and Magic among the Azande.* Oxford: Clarendon Press.

Farmer P. 1993. *AIDS and Accusation: Haiti and the Geography of Blame.* Berkeley: University of California Press.

———. 1999. Hidden epidemics of tuberculosis. In Infectious Diseases and Social Inequality in Latin America: From Hemispheric Insecurity to Global Cooperation. Latin American Program, Working Paper Series no. 239. Pp. 31–55. Washington, DC: Woodrow Wilson International Center for Scholars.

———. 1999. *Infections and Inequalities: The Modern Plagues.* Berkeley: University of California Press.

———. 2003. *Pathologies of Power: Health, Human Rights, and the New War on the Poor.* Berkeley: University of California Press.

Farquhar J. W., N. Maccoby, P. D. Wood, J. K. Alexander, H. Breitrose, B. W. Brown Jr., W. L. Haskell, A. L. McAlister, A. J. Meyer, J. D. Nash, and M. P. Stern. 1977. Community education for cardiovascular health. *Lancet* 1:1192–1195.

Ferguson S. A., D. F. Preusser, A. K. Lund, P. L. Zador, and R. G. Ulmer. 1995. Daylight saving time and motor vehicle crashes: the reduction in pedestrian and vehicle occupant fatalities. *American Journal of Public Health* 85:92–95.

Fernández-Marina R. 1961. The Puerto Rican Syndrome. *Psychiatry* 24:79–82.

Fikree F. F., R. H. Gray, and F. Shah. 1993. Can men be trusted? A comparison of pregnancy histories reported by husbands and wives. *American Journal of Epidemiology* 138:237–242.

First Nations and Inuit Regional Health Survey National Steering Committee. 1999. First Nations and Inuit Regional Health Survey National Report. Available online at: http://www.afn.ca/Programs/Health%20Secretariat/PDF's/title.pdf. Accessed September 2001.

Fleck A. C. and F. A. J. Ianni. 1958. Epidemiology and anthropology: some suggested affinities in theory and method. *Human Organization* 16:38–40.

Fortin J. M., L. K. Hirota, B. E. Bond, A. M. O'Connor, and N. F. Col. 2001. Identifying patient preferences for communicating risk estimates: a descriptive pilot study. *BMC Medical Informatics and Decision Making* 1:2. Available online at: http:www.biomedcentral.com/1472–6947/1/2.

Fortmann S. P. and A. N. Varady. 2000. Effects of a community-wide health education program on cardiovascular disease morbidity and mortality: the Stanford Five-City Project. *American Journal of Epidemiology* 152:316–323.

Fortmann S. P., J. A. Flora, M. A. Winkleby, C. Schooler, C. B. Taylor, and J. W. Farquhar. 1995. Community intervention trials: reflections on the Stanford Five-City Project experience. *American Journal of Epidemiology* 142:576–586.

Foucault M. 1973. *The Birth of the Clinic. An Archaeology of Medical Perception.* A. M. Sheridan Smith, trans. New York: Vintage Books.

Frankel S., C. Davison, and G. Davey Smith. 1991. Lay epidemiology and the rationality of responses to health education. *British Journal of General Practice* 41:428–30.

Frankenberg R. 1988. Risks: corporeal, somatic or incarnate? Responses: natural, clinical or social? Unpublished manuscript. University of Keele, UK: Centre for Medical Social Anthropology.

———. 1993. Risk: Anthropological and Epidemiological Narratives of Prevention. In *Knowledge, Power, and Practice: The Anthropology of Medicine in Everyday Life.* S. Lindenbaum and M Lock, eds. Pp. 219–242. Berkeley: University of California Press.

Fraser W., R. H. Usher, F. H. McLean, C. Bossenberry, M. E. Thomson, M. S. Kramer, L. P. Smith, and H. Power. 1987. Temporal variation in rates of cesarean section for dystocia: does "convenience" play a role? *American Journal of Obstetrics and Gynecology* 156:300–304.

Frenk J., T. Frejka, J. L. Bobadilla, C. Stern, R. Lozano, J. Sepulveda, and M. Jose. 1991. La transición epidemiológica en America Latina [The epidemiologic transition in Latin America]. *Boletin de la Oficina Sanitaria Panamericana* 111:485–496.

Gall N. 1993. *The Death Threat, Part of a Broader Study of Chronic Inflation as Systemic Failure: Latin America and the Polarization of the World Economy.* São Paulo: Fernand Braudel Institute of World Economics.

Gallerani M., R. Manfredini, L. Ricci, E. Grandi, R. Cappato, G. Calo, P. L. Pareschi, and C. Fersini. 1992. Sudden death from pulmonary thromboembolism: chronobiological aspects. *European Heart Journal* 13:661–665.

Galton Francis. 1872. A statistical inquiry into the efficacy of prayer. *Fortnightly Review, New Series* 12:125–135.

García Márquez G. 1989. *Love in the Time of Cholera.* Edith Grossman, trans. New York: Penguin Books.

Geertz, C. 1973. *The Interpretation of Cultures.* New York: Basic Books.

Geiger H. J. 1971. A Health Center in Mississippi – A Case Study in Social Medicine. In *Medicine in a Changing Society.* L. Corey, S. E. Saltman, and M. F. Epstein, eds. Pp. 157–167. St. Louis: C. V. Mosby.

———. 1984. Community Health Centers: Health Care as an Instrument of Social Change. In *Reforming Medicine: Lessons of the Past Quarter Century.* V. W. Sidel and R. Sidel, eds. Pp. 11–32. New York: Pantheon Books.

———. 1993. Community-oriented primary care: the legacy of Sidney Kark. *American Journal of Public Health* 83:946–947.

Gettleman J. 2002. Setting course for adventure, with Imodium. *New York Times,* December 8:A37.

Gibbs W. W. 1995. Lost science in the Third World. *Scientific American* 273:76–83.

Gifford S. M. 1986. The Meaning of Lumps: A Case Study of the Ambiguities of Risk. In *Anthropology and Epidemiology.* C. R. Janes, S. M. Gifford, and R. Stall, eds. Pp. 213–246. Dordrecht, The Netherlands: D. Reidel Publishing.

Gilman R. H., G. S. Marquis, G. Ventura, M. Campos, W. Spira, and F. Diaz. 1993. Water cost and availability: key determinants of family hygiene in a Peruvian shantytown. *American Journal of Public Health* 83:1554–1558.

Glass R. I. and R. E. Black. 1992. The Epidemiology of Cholera. In *Cholera.* D. Barua and W. B. Greenough, eds. Pp. 129–154. New York: Plenum.

Global Task Force on Cholera Control. 1993. Guidelines for cholera control. Revised 1992. WHO/CDD/SER PO4 REV3 1992. Geneva: World Health Organization (WHO).

Good B. J. 1997. Studying mental illness in context: local, global, or universal? *Ethos* 25:230–248.

Goodman, A. H. 1997. Bred in the Bone? *Sciences* 37:20–25.

Goodnough A. 1998. Tracking cancer as never before. *New York Times,* April 26:A30.

Gordon J. E. 1953. Evolution of an Epidemiology of Health, Parts I, II, and III. In *The Epidemiology of Health.* I. Galdston, ed. Pp. 24–73. New York: New York Academy of Medicine.

———. 1958. Medical ecology and the public health. *American Journal of the Medical Sciences* 235:336–359.

Goszczynska M., T. Tyszka, and P. Slovic. 1991. Risk perception in Poland: a comparison with three other countries. *Journal of Behavioral Decision Making* 4:179–193.

Gottschang S. Z. 2000. Reforming Routines: A Baby-Friendly Hospital in Urban China. In *Global Health Policy, Local Realities.* L. M. Whiteford and L. Manderson, eds. Pp. 265–287. Boulder: Lynne Rienner Publishers.

Gotuzzo E., J. Cieza, L. Estremadoyro, and C. Seas. 1994. Cholera: lessons from the epidemic in Peru. *Infectious Disease Clinics of North America* 8:183–205.

Government of South Africa. 2001. South Africa: Evaluation of the New Death Notification Form [BI 1663]. Available online at: http://www.doh.gov.za/nhis/vital/docs/evaluation/sec3.html. Accessed January 2003.

Granovetter M. 1978. Threshold models of collective behavior. *American Journal of Sociology* 83:1420–1443.

Green L. A., G. E. Fryer, B. P. Yawn, D. Lanier, and S. M. Dovey. 2001. The ecology of medical care revisited. *New England Journal of Medicine* 344:2021–2025.

Green L. W. and M. W. Kreuter. 2000. Commentary on the emerging Guide to Community Preventive Services from a health promotion perspective. *American Journal of Preventative Medicine* 18:7–9.

Greenberg M. and D. Wartenberg. 1990. Understanding mass media coverage of disease clusters. *American Journal of Epidemiology* 132:S192–S195.

Guarnaccia P. J. and L. H. Rogler. 1999. Research on culture-bound syndromes: new directions. *American Journal of Psychiatry* 156:1322–1327.

Guarnaccia P. J., G. Canino, M. Rubio-Stipec, and M. Bravo. 1993. The prevalence of *ataques de nervios* in the Puerto Rico disaster study: the role of culture in psychiatric epidemiology. *Journal of Nervous and Mental Disease* 181:157–165.

Guillemin J. 1999. *Anthrax: The Investigation of a Deadly Outbreak.* Berkeley: University of California Press.

Hahn R. A. 1992. The state of federal health statistics on racial and ethnic groups. *Journal of the American Medical Association* 267:268–271.

———. 1995. *Sickness and Healing: An Anthropological Perspective.* New Haven, CT: Yale University Press.

———. 1999. How anthropology can enhance public health practice. In *Anthropology in Public Health: Bridging Differences in Culture and Society.* R. A. Hahn, ed. Oxford: Oxford University Press.

Hahn R. A., B. I. Truman, and N. D. Barker. 1995. Identifying ancestry: the reliability of ancestral identification in the United States by self, proxy, interviewer, and funeral director. *Epidemiology* 7:75–80.

Hahn R. A. and D. F. Stroup. 1994. Race and ethnicity in public health surveillance: criteria for the scientific use of social categories. *Public Health Reports* 109:7–15.

Hahn R. A., J. Mulinare, and S. M. Teutsch. 1992. Inconsistencies in coding of race and ethnicity between birth and death in US infants: a new look at infant mortality, 1983 through 1985. *Journal of the American Medical Association* 267:259–263.

Hall R. L., K. Lopez, and E. Lichtenstein. 1999. A Policy Approach to Reducing Cancer Risk in Northwest Indian Tribes. In *Anthropology in Public Health.* R. Hahn, ed. Pp. 142–162. New York: Oxford University Press.

Hanenberg R. and W. Rojanapithayakorn. 1996. Prevention as policy: how Thailand reduced STD and HIV transmission. *AIDScaptions* 3:24–27.

Harr J. 1996. *A Civil Action.* New York: Vintage Books.

Harwood A. 1977. *Rx: Spiritist as Needed: A Study of a Puerto Rican Community Mental Health Resource.* New York: Wiley.

Hauser W. A. and L. T. Kurland. 1975. The epidemiology of epilepsy in Rochester, Minnesota, 1935 through 1967. *Epilepsia* 16:1–66.

Helliwell T. 2001. Letter: Need for patient consent for cancer registration creates logistical nightmare. *British Medical Journal* 322:730.

Hermida J., C. Laspina, and F. Idrovo. 1994. *Improving Quality of Cholera Case Management in a Hospital Setting in Ecuador.* Bethesda: Quality Assurance Project.

Hicks G. J., J. W. Davis, and R. A. Hicks. 1998. Fatal alcohol-related traffic crashes increase subsequent to changes to and from daylight savings time. *Perceptual and Motor Skills* 86(3 Pt 1):879–882.

Hippocrates. 1957. Airs Waters Places. In *Hippocrates, with an English Translation.* W. H. S. Jones, trans. Pp. 71–137. Cambridge: Harvard University Press.

Holmes O. W., Sr. 1860. Currents and Counter-Currents in Medical Science. An Address delivered before the Massachusetts Medical Society, at the Annual Meeting, May 30, 1860. In *Medical Essays 1842–1882.* Urbana, IL: Project Gutenberg. Available online at: ftp://ibiblio.org/pub/docs/books/gutenberg/etext01/medic10.txt.

Horwitz R. I. and E. C. Yu. 1985. Problems and proposals for interview data in epidemiological research. *International Journal of Epidemiology* 14:463–467.

Hughes C. C., M. A. Tremblay, R. N. Rapoport, and A. H. Leighton. 1960. *People of Cove and Woodlot: Communities from the Viewpoint of Social Psychiatry.* New York: Basic Books.

Inhorn M. C. 1995. Medical anthropology and epidemiology: divergences or convergences? *Social Science and Medicine* 40:285–290.

Inhorn M. C. and K. L. Whittle. 2001. Feminism meets the "new" epidemiologies: toward an appraisal of antifeminist biases in epidemiological research on women's health. *Social Science and Medicine* 53:553–567.

Instituto Nacional de Estadística Geografía e Informática [National Institute of Statistics, Geography and Informatics]. 2003. *Síntesis Metodológica de las Estadísticas Vitales.* [Methodological Synthesis of Vital Statistics]. Mexico City: July. Available online at: http://www.inegi.gob.mx/est/contenidos/espanol/metodologias/registros/sociales/sm_ev.pdf. Accessed May 2004.

Janes C. R. 1990. *Migration, Social Change, and Health: A Samoan Community in Urban California.* Stanford: Stanford University Press.

Janes C. R. and G. M. Ames. 1992. Ethnographic explanations for the clustering of attendance, injury, and health problems in a heavy machinery assembly plant. *Journal of Occupational Medicine* 34:993–1003.

Jones C. P. 2001. Invited commentary: "race," racism, and the practice of epidemiology. *American Journal of Epidemiology* 154:299–306.

Joralemon D. 1998. *Exploring Medical Anthropology.* New York: Allyn and Bacon.

Justice J. 1999. Neglect of Cultural Knowledge in Health Planning: Nepal's Assistant Nurse-Midwife Program. In *Anthropology in Public Health.* R. Hahn, ed. Pp. 327–344. New York: Oxford University Press.

Kark S. L. 1951. Health Centre Service. In *Social Medicine.* E. H. Cluver, ed. Pp. 661–700. South Africa: Central News Agency.

———. 1974. *Epidemiology and Community Medicine.* New York: Appleton.

———. 1981. *The Practice of Community-Oriented Primary Health Care.* New York: Appleton-Century-Crofts.

Kark S. L. and E. Kark. 1962. A Practice of Social Medicine. In *A Practice of Social Medicine*. S. L. Kark and G. W. Steuart, eds. Pp. 3–40. Edinburgh: E. & S. Livingstone.

———. 1981. Community Health Care in a Rural African Population. In *A Practice of Community-Oriented Primary Care*. S. L. Kark, ed. Pp. 194–213. New York: Appleton-Century-Crofts.

Kark S. L. and G. W. Steuart, eds. 1962. *A Practice of Social Medicine. A South African Team's Experiences in Different African Communities*. Edinburgh: E. & S. Livingstone.

Kaufman J. S. and R. S. Cooper. 2001. Commentary: considerations for use of racial/ethnic classification in etiologic research. *American Journal of Epidemiology* 154:291–298.

Kawachi I., B. P. Kennedy, K. Lochner, and D. Prothrow-Stith. 1997. Social capital, income inequality, and mortality. *American Journal of Public Health* 87: 1491–1498.

Kawachi I., B. P. Kennedy, and R. G. Wilkinson. 1999. *The Society and Population Health Reader. Volume I: Income Inequality and Health*. New York: The New Press.

Kendall C. 1989. The Use and Non-use of Anthropology: The Diarrheal Disease Control Program in Honduras. In *Making Our Research Useful: Case Studies in the Utilization of Anthropological Knowledge*. J. van Willigen, B. Rylko-Bauer, and A. McElroy, eds. Pp. 283–303. Boulder: Westview Press.

———. 1990. Public Health and the Domestic Domain: Lessons from Anthropological Research on Diarrheal Diseases. In *Anthropology and Primary Health Care*. J. Coreil and J. D. Mull, eds. Pp. 173–195. Boulder: Westview.

Kilborn P. T. 1998. Black Americans trailing whites in health, studies say. *New York Times*, January 26:A16.

Kirkwood B. R., S. N. Cousens, C. G. Victora, and I. de Zoysa. 1997. Issues in the design and interpretation of studies to evaluate the impact of community-based interventions. *Tropical Medicine and International Health* 2:1022–1029.

Kleinman A., L. Eisenberg, and B. Good. 1978. Culture, illness, and care: clinical lessons from anthropologic and cross-cultural research. *Annals of Internal Medicine* 88:251–258.

Klinenberg E. 2002. *Heat Wave: A Social Autopsy of Disaster in Chicago*. Chicago: University of Chicago Press.

Klovdahl A. S., E. A. Graviss, A. Yaganehdoost, M. W. Ross, G. J. Adams, and J. M. Musser. 2001. Networks and tuberculosis: an undetected community outbreak involving public places. *Social Science and Medicine* 52:681–694.

Kluckhohn C. 1949. *Mirror for Man*. New York: Whittlesey.

Kolata G. 1999. *Flu: The Story of the Great Influenza Pandemic of 1918 and the Search for the Virus That Caused It*. New York: Farrar, Straus, and Giroux.

Kompier M. A., B. Aust, A. M. van den Berg, and J. Siegrist. 2000. Stress prevention in bus drivers: evaluation of 13 natural experiments. *Journal of Occupational Health and Psychology* 5:11–31.

Koopman J. S. and I. M. Longini Jr. 1994. The ecological effects of individual exposures and nonlinear disease dynamics in populations. *American Journal of Public Health* 84:836–842.

Kosek M., C. Bern, and R. L. Guerrant. 2003. The global burden of diarrhoeal disease, as estimated from studies published between 1992 and 2000. *Bulletin of the World Health Organization* 81:197–204.

Krieger N. 1994. Epidemiology and the web of causation: has anyone seen the spider? *Social Science and Medicine* 39:887–903.

———. 2001. Theories for social epidemiology in the 21st century: an ecosocial perspective. *International Journal of Epidemiology* 30:668–677.

Krieger N., D. R. Williams, and N. E. Moss. 1997. Measuring social class in U.S. public health research: concepts, methodologies, and guidelines. *Annual Review of Public Health* 18:341–378.

Kulynych J. and D. Korn. 2002. The effect of the new federal medical-privacy rule on research. *New England Journal of Medicine* 346:201–204.

Kunitz S. J. 1994. *Disease and Social Diversity*. London: Oxford University Press.

Lancet. 1993. Editorial: Do epidemiologists cause epidemics? 341:993–994.

Landsbergis P. A., J. Cahill, and P. Schnall. 1999. The impact of lean production and related new systems of work organization on worker health. *Journal of Occupational Health Psychology* 4:108–130.

Lange C. H. 1965. Culture Change. In *Biennial Review of Anthropology.* B. J. Siegel, ed. Stanford: Stanford University Press.

Law S. P. 1986. The regulation of menstrual cycle and its relationship to the moon. *Acta Obstetricia et Gynecologica Scandinavica* 65:45–48.

Lawlor D. A., S. Frankel, M. Shaw, S. Ebrahim, and G. Davey Smith. 2003. Smoking and ill health: does lay epidemiology explain the failure of smoking cessation programs among deprived populations? *American Journal of Public Health* 93:266–270.

LeClere F. B., R. G. Rogers, and K. Peters. 1998. Neighborhood social context and racial differences in women's heart disease mortality. *Journal of Health and Social Behavior* 39:91–107.

Lefley H. P. 1979. Prevalence of potential falling-out cases among the Black, Latin, and non-Latin White populations of the city of Miami. *Social Science and Medicine* 13B:113–114.

Legator M. S. and S. F. Strawn, eds. 1993. *Chemical Alert!: A Community Action Handbook.* Austin: University of Texas Press.

Legator M. S., B. L. Harper, and M. J. Scott, eds. 1985. *The Health Detective's Handbook: A Guide to the Investigation of Environmental Health Hazards by Nonprofessionals.* Baltimore: The Johns Hopkins University Press.

Leighton A. H. and J. M. Murphy. 1997. Nature of pathology: the character of danger implicit in functional impairment. *Canadian Journal of Psychiatry* 42:714–721.

Leighton D. C., J. S. Harding, D. B. Macklin, A. M. Macmillan, and A. H. Leighton. 1963. *The Character of Danger: Psychiatric Symptoms in Selected Communities.* New York: Basic Books.

Levin J. S. 1996. How religion influences morbidity and health: reflections on natural history, salutogenesis and host resistance. *Social Science and Medicine* 43:849–864.

Levine M. M. and O. S. Levine. 1994. Changes in human ecology and behavior in relation to the emergence of diarrheal diseases, including cholera. *Proceedings of the National Academy of Sciences USA* 91:2390–2394.

Lewontin R. C. 1972. Apportionment of human diversity. *Evolutionary Biology* 6:381–398.

Lilienfeld A. M. and D. E. Lilienfeld. 1980. *Foundations of Epidemiology.* 2nd edition. New York: Oxford University Press.

Lilienfeld J. and S. Graham. 1958. Validity of determining circumcision status by questionnaire as related to epidemiological studies of cancer of the cervix. *Journal of the National Cancer Institute* 21:713–720.

Lindenbaum S. 1979. *Kuru Sorcery: Disease and Danger in the New Guinea Highlands.* New York: Mayfield Publishing.

———. 2001. Kuru, Prions, and human affairs: thinking about epidemics. *Annual Review of Anthropology* 30:363–385.

Lock M. 2001. *Twice Dead: Organ Transplants and the Remaking of Death.* Berkeley: University of California Press.

Loomis D., S. W. Marshall, S. H. Wolf, C. W. Runyan, and J. D. Butts. 2002. Effectiveness of safety measures recommended for prevention of workplace homicide. *Journal of the American Medical Association* 287:1011–1017.

Low S. M. 1985. Culturally interpreted symptoms or culture-bound syndromes: a cross-cultural review of nerves. *Social Science and Medicine* 21:187–196.

Löwy I. 2000. Trustworthy knowledge and desperate patients: clinical tests for new drugs from cancer to AIDS. In *Living and Working with the New Medical Technologies.* M. Lock, Y. Young, and A. Cambrosio, eds. Pp. 49–81. Cambridge: Cambridge University Press.

Lupton D. 1999. *Risk.* New York: Routledge.

Macintyre S., A. Ellaway, and S. Cummins. 2002. Place effects on health: how can we conceptualise, operationalise, and measure them? *Social Science and Medicine* 55:125–139.

Macintyre S., S. MacIver, and A. Sooman. 1993. Area, class and health: should we be focusing on places or people? *Journal of Social Policy* 22:213–234.

Magnusson A. 2000. An overview of epidemiological studies on seasonal affective disorder. *Acta Psychiatrica Scandinavica* 101:176–184.

Management Sciences for Health. 2004. Cultural Groups: Introduction. *The Provider's Guide to Quality and Culture.* Available online at: http://erc.msh.org. Accessed March 2002 and June 2004.

Marmot M. G., G. Davey Smith, S. A. Stansfeld, C. Patel, F. North, J. Head, I. White, E. Brunner, and A. Feeney. 1991. Health inequalities among British civil servants: the Whitehall II Study. *Lancet* 337:1387–1393.

Marmot M. G. and S. L. Syme. 1976. Acculturation and coronary heart disease in Japanese-Americans. *American Journal of Epidemiology* 104:225–247.

May J. M. 1978. History, definition, and problems of medical geography: a general review. (Report to the Commission on Medical Geography of the International Geographical Union, 1952.) *Social Science and Medicine* 12D: 211–219.

Mays V. M., N. A. Ponce, D. L. Washington, and S. D. Cochran. 2003. Classification of race and ethnicity: implications for public health. *Annual Review of Public Health* 24:83–110.

McKinlay J. 1974. A Case for Refocusing Upstream – the Political Economy of Illness. In *Applying Behavioral Science to Cardiovascular Disease Risk.* Proceedings of the American Heart Association Conference. Seattle, Washington.

_____. 1993. The promotion of health through planned sociopolitical change: challenges for research and policy. *Social Science and Medicine* 36:109–117.

McNeil B. J., S. G. Pauker, H. C. Sox Jr., and A. Tversky. 1982. On the elicitation of preferences for alternative therapies. *New England Journal of Medicine* 306:1259–1262.

Melander H., J. Ahlqvist-Rastad, G. Meijer, and B. Beerman 2003. Evidence-b(i)ased medicine – selective reporting from studies sponsored by the pharmaceutical industry: review of studies in new drug applications. *British Medical Journal* 326:1171–1175.

Ministerio de Salud [Ministry of Health] Argentina. 2001. *Modelos de formularios e instructivos del sistema de estadísticas vitales* [Models of Forms and Instructions of the Vital Statistics Program]. Buenos Aires, Argentina: Dirección de Estadística e Información de Salud, Programa Nacional de Estadísticas de Salud [Directorate of Health Statistics and Information, National Program for Health Statistics].

Moerman D. 2002. *Meaning, Medicine, and the "Placebo Effect."* Cambridge: Cambridge University Press.

Moffatt S., P. Phillimore, E. Hudson, and D. Downey. 2000. "Impact? What impact?" Epidemiological research findings in the public domain: a case study from northeast England. *Social Science and Medicine* 51:1755–1769.

Morgan L. 1998. Latin American social medicine and the politics of theory. In *Building a New Biocultural Synthesis: Political-Economic Perspectives in Biological Anthropology.* A. Goodman and T. Leathmann, eds. Pp. 407–424. Ann Arbor: University of Michigan Press.

Morgan M. G., B. Fischhoff, A. Bostrom, and C. J. Atman. 2002. *Risk Communication: A Mental Models Approach.* Cambridge: Cambridge University Press.

Morris M. 1993. Epidemiology and social networks: modeling structural diffusion. *Sociological Methods and Research* 22:99–126.

Morris R. J. 1976. *Cholera 1832: The Social Response to an Epidemic.* London: Croom Helm.

Mullan F. 1982. Community-oriented primary care. An agenda for the '80s. *New England Journal of Medicine* 307:1076–1078.

Murphy J. M. 1994a. Anthropology and psychiatric epidemiology. *Acta Psychiatrica Scandinavica* Supplementum 385:48–57.

_____. 1994b. The Stirling County Study: then and now. In *Special Issue on Psychiatric Epidemiology, International Review of Psychiatry* 6:329–348. S. B. Guze and W. M. Compton, eds.

Murphy J. M., N. M. Laird, R. R. Monson, A. M. Sobol, and A. H. Leighton. 2000. A 40-year perspective on the prevalence of depression: the Stirling County Study. *Archives of General Psychiatry* 57:209–215.

Nadel S. F. 1957. *A Theory of Social Structure.* London: Cohen and West.

Nakamura J. W., C. R. McLeod, and J. F. McDermott Jr. 1994. Temporal variation in adolescent suicide attempts. *Suicide and Life-threatening Behavior* 24:343–349.

Nash J. and M. Kirsch. 1986. Polychlorinated biphenyls in the electrical machinery industry: an ethnological study of community action and corporate responsibility. *Social Science and Medicine* 23:131–138.

Nastasi B. K. and M. J. Berg. 1999. Using ethnography to strengthen and evaluate intervention programs. In *Using Ethnographic Data. Volume Seven in The Ethnographer's Toolkit.* J. Schensul and M. D. LeCompte, eds. Pp. 1–56. Walnut Creek, CA: Alta Mira Press.

National Center for Health Statistics. 2001. Health Interview Health Measures in the New 1997 Redesigned National Health Interview Survey. Available online at: www.cdc.gov/nchs/about/major/nhis/hisdesgn.htm. Accessed September 2001.

———. 2003. *Revisions of the U.S. Standard Certificates of Death.* National Vital Statistics System. November. Available online at: http://www.cdc. gov/nchs/data/dvs/DEATH11-03final-ACC.pdf. Accessed May 2004.

Nations M. K. 1986. Epidemiological Research on Infectious Disease: Quantitative Rigor or Rigormortis? Insights from Ethnomedicine. In *Anthropology and Epidemiology: Interdisciplinary Approaches to the Study of Health and Disease.* C. R. Janes, R. Stall, and S. Gifford, eds. Pp. 97–123. Dordrecht, The Netherlands: Reidel.

Nations M. K. and M. L. Amaral. 1991. Flesh, blood, souls, and households: cultural validity in mortality inquiry. *Medical Anthropology Quarterly* 5:204–220.

Nations M. K. and C. M. G. Monte. 1996. "I'm not dog, no!": cries of resistance against cholera control campaigns. *Social Science and Medicine* 43:1007–1024.

Nations M. K., M. A. de Sousa, L. L. Correia, and D. M. da Silva. 1988. Brazilian popular healers as effective promoters of oral rehydration therapy (ORT) and related child survival strategies. *Bulletin of the Pan American Health Organization* 22:335–354.

Negre J. 1985. Colors, races, languages, and diseases. *Journal of the American Medical Association* 254:1310.

Nguyen V-K. and K. Peschard. 2003. Anthropology, inequality, and disease: a review. *Annual Review of Anthropology* 32:447–474.

Nichter M. 1993. Social science lessons from diarrhea research and their application to ARI. *Human Organization* 52:53–67.

Nichter M., N. Vuckovic, G. Quintero, and C. Ritenbaugh. 1997. Smoking experimentation and initiation among adolescent girls: qualitative and quantitative findings. *Tobacco Control* 6:285–295.

O'Neil J. D., J. R. Reading, and A. Leader. 1998. Changing the relations of surveillance: the development of a discourse of resistance in aboriginal epidemiology. *Human Organization* 57:230–237.

Oakley A. 1998. Experimentation and social interventions: a forgotten but important history. *British Medical Journal* 317:1239–1242.

Oppenheimer G. M. and D. Rosner. 2002. Two lives, three legs, one journey: a retrospective appreciation of Zena Stein and Mervyn Susser. *International Journal of Epidemiology* 31:49–53.

Oths K. S. 1998. Assessing variation in health status in the Andes: a biocultural model. *Social Science and Medicine* 47:1017–1030.

Pan American Health Organization. 1995. Summary of reported cholera cases and deaths by subregion and country 1991–1995. *Cholera Situation in the Americas Update Number 13.* Washington, DC: Pan American Health Organization.

Panum P. L. 1940. *Observations Made during the Epidemic of Measles on the Faroe Islands in the Year 1846.* New York: Delta Omega Society.

Paredes P., M. de la Peña, E. Flores-Guerra, J. Diaz, and J. Trostle. 1996. Factors influencing physicians' prescribing behaviour in the treatment of childhood diarrhoea: knowledge may not be the clue. *Social Science and Medicine* 42:1141–1153.

Paredes P. J., B. A. Yeager, and C. F. Lanata. 1992. Children with persistent diarrhoea. *Lancet* 339:1236–1237.

Parker R. G., D. Easton, and C. H. Klein. 2000. Structural barriers and facilitators in HIV prevention: a review of international research. *AIDS* 14 (Suppl 1): S22–S32.

Parsons T. 1975. The sick role and the role of the physician reconsidered. *Milbank Memorial Fund Quarterly: Health and Society* 53:257–278.

Paul B. D., ed. 1955. *Health, Culture, and Community: Case Studies of Public Reactions to Health Programs.* New York: Russell Sage Foundation.

Payer L. 1988. *Medicine and Culture: Varieties of Treatment in the United States, England, West Germany, and France.* New York: Henry Holt.

Paz O. 1993 [1950]. *El Laberinto de la Soledad* (The Labyrinth of Solitude) 2nd edition. Mexico City: Fondo de Cultura Económica.

Peckova M., C. E. Fahrenbruch, L. A. Cobb, and A. P. Hallstrom. 1999. Weekly and seasonal variation in the incidence of cardiac arrests. *American Heart Journal* 137:512–515.

Petersen D. J. and G. R. Alexander. 1992. Seasonal variation in adolescent conceptions, induced abortions, and late initiation of prenatal care. *Public Health Reports* 107:701–706.

Petrera M. and M. Montoya. 1993. *Impacto económico de la epidemia del cólera* [The economic impact of the Cholera epidemic]. *Perú 1991. Programa de políticas de salud, Serie informes técnicos* [Health Policy Program, Technical Report] No. 22 April. Washington, DC: Pan American Health Organization.

Pezdek K. and W. P. Banks, eds. 1996. *The Recovered Memory/False Memory Debate.* San Diego: Academic Press.

Phillips D. P., C. A. Van Voorhees, and T. E. Ruth. 1992. The birthday: lifeline or deadline? *Psychosomatic Medicine* 54:532–542.

Polgar S. 1962. Health and human behavior: areas of interest common to the social and medical sciences. *Current Anthropology* 3:159–205.

———. 1963. Health action in cross-cultural perspective. In *Handbook of Medical Sociology.* H. E. Freeman, S. Levine, and L. G. Reeder, eds. Pp. 397–419. Englewood Cliffs, NJ: Prentice-Hall.

Portaluppi F., R. Manfredini, and C. Fersini. 1999. From a static to a dynamic concept of risk: the circadian epidemiology of cardiovascular events. *Chronobiology International* 16:33–49.

Prashad V. 1994. Native dirt/imperial ordure: the cholera of 1832 and the morbid resolutions of modernity. *Journal of Historical Sociology* 7:243–260.

Prideaux D. 2002. Editorial: Researching the outcomes of educational interventions: a matter of design. *British Medical Journal* 324:126–127.

Puska P., E. Vartiainen, J. Tuomilehto, V. Salomaa, and A. Nissinen. 1998. Changes in premature deaths in Finland: successful long-term prevention of cardiovascular diseases. *Bulletin of the World Health Organization* 76:419–425.

Rabbani G. H. and W. B. Greenough. 1992. Pathophysiology and clinical aspects of cholera. In *Cholera*. D. Barua and W. B. Greenough, eds. Pp. 209–228. New York: Plenum.

Radda K. E., J. J. Schensul, W. B. Disch, J. A. Levy, and C. Y. Reyes. 2003. Assessing human immunodeficiency virus (HIV) risk among older urban adults: a model for community-based research partnership. *Family and Community Health* 26:203–213.

Rapp R. 1998. Refusing prenatal diagnosis: the uneven meanings of bioscience in a multicultural world. In *Cyborg Babies: From Techno-Sex to Techno Tots*. R. Davis-Floyd and J. Dumit, eds. Pp. 143–167. New York: Routledge.

———. 1999. *Testing Women, Testing the Fetus: The Social Impact of Amniocentesis in America*. New York: Routledge.

Rapp R., D. Heath, and K.-S. Taussig. 2001. Genealogical dis-ease: where hereditary abnormality, biomedical explanation, and family responsibility meet. In *Relative Values: Reconfiguring Kinship Studies*. S. Franklin and S. McKinnon, eds. Pp. 384–409. Durham: Duke University Press.

Redelmeier, D. A. and A. Tversky. 1990. Discrepancy between medical decisions for individual patients and for groups. *New England Journal of Medicine* 322: 1162–1164.

Reeler A. V. 2000. Anthropological perspectives on injections: a review. *Bulletin of the World Health Organization* 78:135–143.

Reingold A. L. 1998. Outbreak investigations – a perspective. *Emerging Infectious Diseases* 4:21–27. Available online at: http://www.cdc.gov/ncidod/EID/vol4no1/reingold.htm.

Rogers E. S. 1960. *Human Ecology and Health: An Introduction for Administrators*. New York: Macmillan.

Romer D. and P. Jamieson. 2001a. Advertising, smoker imagery, and the diffusion of smoking behavior. In *Smoking: Risk, Perception, and Policy*. P. Slovic, ed. Pp. 127–155. Thousand Oaks, CA: Sage Publications.

———. 2001b. The role of perceived risk in starting and stopping smoking. In *Smoking: Risk, Perception and Policy*. P. Slovic, ed. Pp. 64–80. Thousand Oaks, CA: Sage Publications.

Ropeik D. and G. Gray. 2002. *Risk: A Practical Guide for Deciding What's Really Safe and What's Really Dangerous in the World Around You*. Boston: Houghton Mifflin.

Rose G. 1985. Sick individuals and sick populations. *International Journal of Epidemiology* 14:32–38.

Rosen G. 1947. What is social medicine? A genetic analysis of the concept. *Bulletin of the History of Medicine* 21:674–733.

———. 1955. Problems in the application of statistical analysis to questions of health: 1700–1880. *Bulletin of the History of Medicine* 29:27–45.

Rosenberg C. E. 1992. *Explaining Epidemics and Other Studies in the History of Medicine*. Cambridge: Cambridge University Press.

Ross C. E. and J. Mirowsky. 1984. Socially desirable response and acquiescence in a cross-cultural survey of mental health. *Journal of Health and Social Behavior* 25:189–197.

Rothman K. J. 1981. The rise and fall of epidemiology, 1950–2000. *New England Journal of Medicine* 304:600–602.

Roueché B. 1947 [1980]. "Eleven Blue Men" from *The Medical Detectives*. Pp. 1–12. New York: Washington Square Press.

Rubel A., C. W. O'Nell, and R. Collado-Ardon. 1984. *Susto: A Folk Illness.* Berkeley: University of California Press.

Rubel A. J. 1964. The epidemiology of a folk illness: Susto in Hispanic America. *Ethnology* 3:268–283.

Sackett D. L. 1979. Bias in analytic research. *Journal of Chronic Diseases* 32:51–63.

Salgado de Snyder V. N., M. J. Diaz-Perez, and V. D. Ojeda. 2000. The prevalence of nervios and associated symptomatology among inhabitants of Mexican rural communities. *Culture, Medicine, and Psychiatry* 24:453–470.

Sattenspiel L. and D. A. Herring. 1998. Structured epidemic models and the spread of influenza in the Norway House District of Manitoba, Canada. *Human Biology* 70:91–115.

Scheper-Hughes N. 1992. *Death Without Weeping: The Violence of Everyday Life in Brazil.* Berkeley: University of California Press.

Schinazi R. B. 2000. The probability of a cancer cluster due to chance alone. *Statistics in Medicine* 19:2195–2198.

Schwartz S., E. Susser, and M. Susser. 1999. A future for epidemiology? *Annual Review of Public Health* 20:15–33.

Scotch N. A. 1960. A preliminary report on the relation of sociocultural factors to hypertension among the Zulu. *Annals of the New York Academy of Sciences* 84:1000–1009.

———. 1963a. Medical Anthropology. In *Biennial Review of Anthropology*. B. J. Siegel, ed. Pp. 30–68. Stanford: Stanford University Press.

———. 1963b. Sociocultural factors in the epidemiology of Zulu hypertension. *American Journal of Public Health* 53:1205–1213.

Scotch N. A. and H. J. Geiger. 1962. The epidemiology of rheumatoid arthritis: a review with special attention to social factors. *Journal of Chronic Diseases* 15:1037–1067.

———. 1963. The epidemiology of essential hypertension: a review with special attention to psychologic and sociocultural factors. *Journal of Chronic Diseases* 16:1183–1213.

Scrimshaw S. C. and E. Hurtado. 1988. Anthropological involvement in the Central American diarrheal disease control project. *Social Science and Medicine* 27:97–105.

Sen A. 1992. Missing women. *British Medical Journal* 304:587–588.

Sepulveda J. 1993. *La salud de los pueblos indigenas de México* [The Health of Indigenous Peoples in Mexico]. México: Secretaría de Salud-Instituto Nacional Indigenista.

Setel P. W. 1999. *A Plague of Paradoxes: AIDS, Culture, and Demography in Northern Tanzania.* Chicago: University of Chicago Press.

Shryock R. H. 1961. The History of Quantification in Medical Science. In *Quantification: A History of the Meaning of Measurement in the Natural and Social Sciences*. H. Woolf, ed. Pp. 85–107. Indianapolis: Bobbs-Merrill.

Shulkin D. J. 1995. The July phenomenon revisited: are hospital complications associated with new house staff? *American Journal of Medical Quality* 10:14–17.

Simonoff J. S. 1997. The "Unusual Episode" and a second statistics course. *Journal of Statistics Education* 5. Available online at: http://www.amstat.org/publications/jse/v5n1/simonoff.html. Accessed March 2001.

Singer M. 2001. Toward a bio-cultural and political economic integration of alcohol, tobacco, and drug studies in the coming century. *Social Science and Medicine* 53:199–213.

———. 2003. The Hispanic Health Council: an experiment in applied anthropology. *Practicing Anthropology* 25:2–7.

Singer M., T. Stopka, C. Siano, et al. 2000. The social geography of AIDS and hepatitis risk: qualitative approaches for assessing local differences in sterile-syringe access among injection drug users. *American Journal of Public Health* 90:1049–1056.

SIPRI: Stockholm International Peace Research Institute. 2002. *SIPRI Yearbook 2002: Armaments, Disarmament, and International Security*. Oxford: Oxford University Press. Tables 6.1 and 6A.3. Available online at: http://projects.sipri.se/milex/mex_wnr_table.html. Accessed June 2003.

Skolbekken J.-A. 1995. The risk epidemic in medical journals. *Social Science and Medicine* 43:291–305.

Slovic P. 1987. Perception of risk. *Science* 236:280–285.

———. 1997. Trust, emotion, sex, politics, and science: surveying the risk assessment battlefield. *The University of Chicago Legal Forum* 1997:59–99.

Smedley B. D. and S. L. Syme, eds. 2000. *Promoting Health: Intervention Strategies from Social and Behavioral Research*. Institute of Medicine. Washington, DC: National Academy Press.

Snow J. 1936 [1855]. *Snow on Cholera; Being a Reprint of Two Papers by John Snow*. 2nd edition. New York: Commonwealth Fund.

Snowdon C., J. Garcia, and D. Elbourne. 1997. Making sense of randomization: responses of parents of critically ill babies to random allocation of treatment in a clinical trial. *Social Science and Medicine* 9:1337–1355.

Sontag S. 1978. *Disease as Metaphor*. New York: Farrar, Straus and Giroux.

———. 1988. *AIDS and Its Metaphors*. New York: Farrar, Straus and Giroux.

Stanton B. F., J. D. Clemens, K. M. A. Aziz, and M. Rahman. 1987. Twenty-four-hour recall, knowledge-attitude-practice questionnaires, and direct observations of sanitary practices: a comparative study. *Bulletin of the World Health Organization* 65:217–222.

Stebbins K. R. 1997. Clearing the air: challenges to introducing smoking restrictions in West Virginia. *Social Science and Medicine* 44:1393–1401.

Stein Z. 1985. A woman's age: childbearing and child rearing. *American Journal of Epidemiology* 121:327–342.

———. 1990. HIV prevention: the need for methods women can use. *American Journal of Public Health* 80:460–462.

Sterne J. A. C. and G. Davey Smith. 2001. Sifting the evidence – what's wrong with significance tests? *British Medical Journal* 322:226–231.

Stone L. and J. G. Campbell. 1984. The use and misuse of surveys in international development: an experiment from Nepal. *Human Organization* 43:27–37.

Suchman L. and B. Jordan. 1990. Interactional troubles in face-to-face survey interviews, and comments. *Journal of the American Statistical Association* 85:232–253.

Susser M. 1973. *Causal Thinking in the Health Sciences: Concepts and Strategies of Epidemiology*. London: Oxford University Press.

———. 1987. Social science and public health. In *Epidemiology, Health, and Society*. Susser M., ed. Pp. 177–185. New York, Oxford: Oxford University Press.

———. 1993. A South African odyssey in community health: a memoir of the impact of the teachings of Sidney Kark. *American Journal of Public Health* 83:1039–1042.

———. 1999. Pioneering community-oriented primary care. *Bulletin of the World Health Organization* 77:436–438.

Susser M. and E. Susser. 1996. Choosing a future for epidemiology: II. From black box to Chinese boxes and eco-epidemiology. *American Journal of Public Health* 86:674–677.

Swerdlow D. L., E. D. Mintz, M. Rodriguez, E. Tejada, C. Ocampo, L. Espejo, T. J. Barrett, J. Petzelt, N. H. Bean, L. Seminario, and R. V. Tauxe. 1994. Severe life-threatening cholera associated with blood group O in Peru: implications for the Latin American epidemic. *Journal of Infectious Diseases* 170:468–472.

Syme S. L. 1974. Behavioral factors associated with the etiology of physical disease: a social epidemiological approach. *American Journal of Public Health* 64:1043–1045.

Tacket C. O., G. Losonsky, J. P. Nataro, S. S. Wasserman, S. J. Cryz, R. Edelman, and M. M. Levine. 1995. Extension of the volunteer challenge model to study South American cholera in a population of volunteers predominantly with blood group antigen O. *Transactions of the Royal Society of Tropical Medicine and Hygiene* 89:75–77.

Takahashi K., M. Washio, A. Ren, N. Tokui, T. C. Aw, and O. Wong. 2001. An international comparison of the involvement of epidemiology in the most frequently cited publications in the field of clinical medicine. *Journal of Epidemiology* 11:41–45.

Talley N. J., A. L. Weaver, A. R. Zinsmeister, and L. J. Melton III. 1994. Self-reported diarrhea: what does it mean? *American Journal of Gastroenterology* 89:1160–1164.

Tapper, M. 1999. *In the Blood: Sickle Cell Anemia and the Politics of Race*. Philadelphia: University of Pennsylvania Press.

Taubes G. 1995. Epidemiology faces its limits. *Science* 269:164–169.

Tauxe R. V., E. D. Mintz, and R. E. Quick. 1995. Epidemic Cholera in the New World: translating field epidemiology into new prevention strategies. *Emerging Infectious Diseases* 1:141–146.

Temkin O. 1971. *The Falling Sickness: A History of Epilepsy from the Greeks to the Beginnings of Modern Neurology*. 2nd rev. edition. Baltimore: The Johns Hopkins University Press.

Terris M. 1962. The scope and methods of epidemiology. *American Journal of Public Health* 52:1371–1376.

———. 1985. The changing relationships of epidemiology and society: the Robert Cruickshank Lecture. *Journal of Public Health Policy* 6:15–36.

Timmermans S. 1995. Cui bono? Institutional review board ethics and ethnographic research. *Studies in Symbolic Interaction* 19:153–173.

Todorov A. and C. Kirchner. 2000. Bias in proxies' reports of disability: data from the National Health Interview Survey on Disability. *American Journal of Public Health* 90:1248–1253.

Tollman S. M. 1994. The Pholela Health Centre – the origins of community-oriented primary health care (COPC). An appreciation of the work of Sidney and Emily Kark. *South African Medical Journal* 84:653–658.

Tolson G. C., J. M. Barnes, G. A. Gay, and L. Kowaleski. 1991. The 1989 revision of the U.S. standard certificates and reports. National Center for Health Statistics. *Vital and Health Statistics*, Series 4, No. 28, pp. 1–31.

Toumey C. P. 1996. *Conjuring Science: Science As Meaning in American Culture.* New Brunswick: Rutgers University Press.

Trostle J. A. 1986a. Anthropology and Epidemiology in the Twentieth Century: A Selective History of Collaborative Projects and Theoretical Affinities, 1920 to 1970. In *Anthropology and Epidemiology: Interdisciplinary Approaches to the Study of Health and Disease.* C. R. Janes, R. Stall, and S. Gifford, eds. Pp. 59–94. Dordrecht, The Netherlands: Reidel.

———. 1986b. Early Work in Anthropology and Epidemiology: From Social Medicine to the Germ Theory, 1840 to 1920. In *Anthropology and Epidemiology: Interdisciplinary Approaches to the Study of Health and Disease.* C. R. Janes, R. Stall, and S. Gifford, eds. Pp. 25–57. Dordrecht, The Netherlands: Reidel.

———. 1987. *Managing Epilepsy: A Community Study of Chronic Illness in Rochester, Minnesota.* Ph.D. Dissertation in Medical Anthropology. University of California, Berkeley and San Francisco.

———. 1996. Introduction: Inappropriate distribution of medicines by professionals in developing countries. *Social Science and Medicine* 42:1117–1120.

———. 2000. Conclusion. International Health Research: The Rules of the Game. In *Global Health Policy, Local Realities: The Fallacy of the Level Playing Field.* L. Whiteford and L. Manderson, eds. Pp. 291–313. Boulder: Lynne Rienner.

Trostle J. and J. Sommerfeld. 1996. Medical anthropology and epidemiology. *Annual Review of Anthropology* 25:253–274.

Trostle J., W. A. Hauser, and F. W. Sharbrough. 1989. Psychologic and social adjustment to epilepsy in Rochester, Minnesota. *Neurology* 39:633–637.

Tufte E. R. 1983. *The Visual Display of Quantitative Information.* Chesire, CT: Graphics Press.

United Nations. 2001. *Principles and Recommendations for a Vital Statistics System Revision 2.* Series M, No.19, Rev. 2. Department of Economic and Social Affairs, Statistics Section. New York: United Nations.

U.S. Bureau of the Census. 2001a. Overview of race and Hispanic origin. U.S. Census Brief. C2KBR/01-1. March 2001. Available online at:

http://www.census.gov/prod/2001pubs/c2kbr01-1.pdf. Accessed September 2002.

———. 2001b. The two or more races population: 2000b. U.S. Census Brief. C2KBR/01-6. November. Available online at: http://www.census.gov/prod/2001pubs/c2kbr01-6.pdf. Accessed September 2002.

United States Government Accounting Office (USGAO). 1983. A troubled project – rural water and environmental sanitation in Peru; report to the Administrator, Agency for International Development. GAO/ID-83-42. Washington, DC: USGAO.

Verdejo G. 1998. Argentina: *Situación de salud y tendencias* [Health Status and Trends], *1986–1995*. Publicación No. 46. Buenos Aires: Organización Panamericana de la Salud.

Verdery K. 1999. *The Political Lives of Dead Bodies*. New York: Columbia University Press.

Victora C. G., S. R. Huttly, S. C. Fuchs, F. C. Barros, M. Garenne, O. Leroy, O. Fontaine, J. P. Beau, V. Fauveau, H. R. Chowdhury, M. Yunus, J. Chakraborty, A. M. Sarder, S. K. Kapoor, M. K. Bhan, L. M. Nath, and J. C. Martines. 1993. International differences in clinical patterns of diarrhoea deaths. *Journal of Diarrhoeal Diseases Research* 11:25–29.

Virchow R. I. 1985. The Epidemics of 1848. In *Collected Essays on Public Health and Epidemiology*. L. J. Rather, ed. Pp. 113–119. Canton, MA: Science History Publications.

Vuckovic N. 1999. Fast relief: buying time with medications. *Medical Anthropology Quarterly* 13:51–68.

Wallinga J., W. J. Edmunds, and M. Kretzschmar. 1999. Perspective: human contact patterns and the spread of airborne infectious diseases. *Trends in Microbiology* 7:372–377.

Wechsler H., N. A. Rigotti, J. Gledhill-Hoyt, and H. Lee. 1998. Increased levels of cigarette use among college students: a cause for national concern. *Journal of the American Medical Association* 280:1673–1678.

Weed, J. A. 1995. Vital statistics in the United States: preparing for the next century. *Population Index* 61:527–539. Available online at: http://popindex.princeton.edu/Articles/Weed.html. Accessed May 2004.

Weidman H. H. 1979. Falling-out: a diagnostic and treatment problem viewed from a transcultural perspective. *Social Science and Medicine* 13B:95–112.

Weiss M. G. 1988. Cultural models of diarrheal illness: conceptual framework and review. *Social Science and Medicine* 27:5–16.

———. 2001. Cultural epidemiology: an introduction and overview. *Anthropology and Medicine* 8:1–29.

Wellin E. 1955. Water Boiling in a Peruvian Town. In *Health, Culture and Community: Case Studies of Public Reactions to Health Programs*. B. D. Paul, ed. Pp. 71–103. New York: Russell Sage Foundation.

Wells G. L., M. Small, S. Penrod, R. S. Malpass, S. M. Fulero, and C. A. E. Brimacombe. 1998. Eyewitness identification procedures: recommendations for lineups and photospreads. *Law and Human Behavior* 22: 603–647.

White K. L. 1997. The ecology of medical care: origins and implications for population-based healthcare research. *Health Services Research* 32:11–21.

White K. L., T. F. Williams, and B. G. Greenburg. 1961. The ecology of medical care. *New England Journal of Medicine* 265:885–892.

White R. 1999. *Putting Risk in Perspective.* Lanham, MD: Rowman & Littlefield.

Wilkinson R. G. 1996. *Unhealthy Societies: The Afflictions of Inequality.* London: Routledge.

Williams D. D. R. and J. Garner. 2002. The case against "the evidence": a different perspective on evidence-based medicine. *British Journal of Psychiatry* 180:8–12.

Williams R. A. 1975. *Textbook of Black-Related Diseases.* New York: McGraw-Hill.

Winch P. J., A. M. Makemba, S. R. Kamazima, G. K. Lwihula, P. Lubega, J. N. Minjas, and C. J. Shiff. 1994. Seasonal variation in the perceived risk of malaria: implications for the promotion of insecticide-impregnated bed nets. *Social Science and Medicine* 39:63–75.

World Bank. 1993. *World Development Report 1993: Investing in Health.* New York: Oxford University Press.

———. 1999. *World Development Report 1998/99: Knowledge for Development.* Washington, DC: International Bank for Reconstruction and Development.

World Health Organization (WHO). 1992. *International Statistical Classification of Diseases and Related Health Problems, 1989 Revision.* (ICD-10). Geneva: World Health Organization.

———. 2000. WHO Report on Global Surveillance of Epidemic-Prone Infectious Diseases. Table 4.1. Cholera, cases and total number of deaths reported to WHO, and number of countries reporting, 1950–1998 – Africa. WHO/CDS/CSR/ ISR/2000.1. Geneva: World Health Organization (WHO). Available online at: http://www.who.int/emc-documents/surveillance/docs/whocdscsrisr2001.pdf/index.html.

Yen I. H. and G. A. Kaplan. 1999a. Neighborhood social environment and risk of death: multilevel evidence from the Alameda County Study. *American Journal of Epidemiology* 149:898–907.

———. 1999b. Poverty area residence and changes in depression and perceived health status: evidence from the Alameda County Study. *International Journal of Epidemiology* 28:90–94.

Yip P. S., J. Lee, and Y. B. Cheung. 2002. The influence of the Chinese zodiac on fertility in Hong Kong SAR. *Social Science and Medicine* 55:1803–1812.

Yoder S. 1995. Examining ethnomedical diagnoses and treatment choices for diarrheal disorders in Lubumbashi Swahili. *Medical Anthropology* 16:211–247.

Index